Nurses' Aids Series

SPECIAL INTEREST TEXT

Gastroenterological Nursing

Helen E. Gribble
SRN, SCM, RNT, MTD, QN

Assistant Director of Nursing Education,
St Bartholomew's School of Nursing (City and Hackney District),
London
Examiner to the General Nursing Council

BAILLIÈRE TINDALL · LONDON

A BAILLIÈRE TINDALL book published by
Cassell & Collier Macmillan Publishers Ltd
35 Red Lion Square, London WC1R 4SG
and at Sydney, Auckland, Toronto, Johannesburg
an affiliate of
Macmillan Publishing Co. Inc.
New York

First published 1977

ISBN 0 7020 0605 X

Printed by Page Bros (Norwich) Ltd,
Mile Cross Lane, Norwich

CONTENTS

Preface

Every year about 325 000 persons in England and Wales are admitted to hospital for investigation and treatment of one of the more common disorders of the gastrointestinal tract, and this figure is small compared with the number who consult their general practitioner for both minor and major conditions. The nurse, whether working in hospital, industry or in the community will therefore often be caring for such sick persons or acting as adviser to their anxious relatives or friends. Her confidence to fulfil this task and her care of her patient will benefit greatly from a proper understanding of the common disorders of the gastrointestinal tract. This book has been written with the needs of the senior student nurse or newly qualified staff nurse very much in mind. It assumes a basic knowledge of anatomy and physiology but sets out to give these in more depth as an understanding of normal function is so essential a part in the appreciation of the abnormal.

The book is divided into fourteen chapters: the majority deal with one particular section of the gastrointestinal tract and explain its development from the embryonic stage, because this helps in an understanding of the congenital anomalies which may occur. The disorders are classified mainly as traumatic, infective, inflammatory and neoplastic, and are explained together with the appropriate diagnostic tests. Treatment is discussed under two main headings, medical and surgical, the latter including a short description of the common operative techniques in use. The first chapter in the book deals with general nursing, giving an overall view of the care required by patients with any gastrointestinal condition, but each subsequent chapter deals with the specific nursing care that is directly related to conditions of that part of the gut. Pharmacology is also to be found in each chapter.

Disorders of the gastrointestinal tract affect children and adults alike and therefore a chapter on paediatric nursing has been included. The final chapter gives details of the preparation and care required by the patient undergoing any of the investigations mentioned in the preceding chapters. It is to be hoped that nurses will enjoy using a textbook which sets out to look at a subject as a whole, progressing from the structure and function of the part to the pathology, diagnosis, treatment and eventual rehabilitation of the patient back into the community. Not every patient will return home, and when one considers that 39 000 persons in this country die each year from a malignant condition of the gut, there are many who will spend the closing weeks of their life in the care of the nurse. I hope this book will give a better awareness of the needs of the terminally ill patient.

Finally, my thanks are due to the many friends and colleagues who have encouraged and advised me on the content of this book, and especially to Rosemary Bailey who has listened to and helped me correct the script. I also owe a debt of gratitude to Baillière Tindall for being so patient.

March 1976   HELEN GRIBBLE

CHAPTER 1

General Nursing Care

Conditions of the gastrointestinal tract give rise to a variety of symptoms. Some people may tolerate these for a considerable while, perhaps buying a mild remedy in the hope that they will soon be better and not require further treatment. In time they may come to realize that skilled care is needed, they may have lost a considerable amount of weight, experienced a chronic blood loss for several weeks or months and find that foods which they once enjoyed no longer stimulate the same pleasure. Reluctantly many will go to see their doctor, often fearing that they will hear bad news, and not being surprised to find that they are referred to hospital for investigation and possible treatment. The thought of undergoing some investigations on the digestive tract will cause many people to be apprehensive, they may consider these to be embarrassing and frankly uncomfortable. The patient may conjure up in his mind many possibilities of treatment that may be required and the idea of swallowing a tube, undergoing an operation and perhaps having a colostomy raised may fill him with anxiety and distaste.

With this background the patient arrives in hospital in the outpatient department. The clinic nurse must appreciate that the patient is bewildered and often frightened of the medical terms which he hears used. He will need a calm and patient approach, to be given sufficient explanation in terms which he can understand and not to be offered too much detail to assimilate all at once. The

1

patient's relatives must also be considered, and many doctors will talk to both patient and relative together, outlining their proposed plan. If admission to hospital is contemplated it is often the practice when arranging this to provide the patient with a booklet containing helpful advice with regard to their stay in hospital. The busy nurse should find time to answer any small queries that the patient may pose, endeavouring to give the impression that she has unlimited time for that particular patient as this will increase his confidence in the staff who will look after him. A talk with the medical social worker may help to allay anxiety and she may also give practical help with regard to the care of dependants at home, finances and problems of employment.

In the ward situation the nurse must maintain this trust and cooperation that has gradually been built up, for this will help the patient through some of the unpleasant procedures which may be necessary. Some treatments may cause embarrassment to the patient and the nurse should maintain a calm and professional approach to put him at ease. The patient may be distressed by vomiting, unpleasant stools or discharges and the nurse should invent ways of dealing with such excretions with as little fuss as possible. Above all, the patient and his relatives must feel that someone cares about him as an individual, and that the prime object of the patient's stay in hospital is a speedy recovery and a return to the family and full capacity as quickly as possible.

ADMISSION TO HOSPITAL

Indications for admission

Conditions of the gastrointestinal tract may require the person to be admitted to hospital at some stage; this may be in order that certain diagnostic tests can be carried out or for definite medical and surgical treatment to be performed. Many investigations can be undertaken when the patient attends the outpatient department, but some tests take place over several hours and involve considerable preparation of the patient, or may require a general anaesthetic with subsequent skilled nursing care in the postanaesthetic period; for these procedures the patient should be admitted to the ward until all tests are complete and a diagnosis has been made.

Following diagnosis of the condition the patient may remain in hospital for medical treatment, being discharged home once relief of symptoms has been achieved, possibly to continue similar care at home for a period before returning to work. In some instances time spent in a medical ward may be to improve the general condition of the patient in order that he is fit to undergo surgery, the patient either being transferred direct to a surgical ward or returning home for a few weeks before readmission for operation. For some patients treatment may take the form of radiotherapy for an inoperable carcinoma, and the period spent in hospital may last several weeks.

Admission procedure

Patients are admitted to the ward either as a planned admission or as result of some emergency which has arisen. The nurse must remember that with the former group, the patient has had some time in which to accustom himself to the idea of being an inpatient, but even so may view his approaching period in hospital with considerable fear and apprehension especially at the thought of numerous tests and investigations to be carried out, some of which may be unpleasant or painful. Two of the predisposing factors to conditions affecting the gastrointestinal tract are those of stress and worry, and an impending stay in hospital is likely to increase the symptoms of the condition for which the patient has been admitted.

For the person who is admitted as an emergency little time has been available for the patient to adjust to the prospect of a period in hospital. In fact many patients may be relieved at the idea of being admitted for treatment even if this is likely to involve surgery, as they can see an end to the pain and distress which they may have experienced for the past few hours or days. Even so, sudden admission may result from collapse at work or when travelling and the patient may find himself in a hospital some way from home; the nurse should remember that prompt contact with relatives, making facilities available for them to visit, will do much to allay anxiety for both the patient and his family.

Some patients will require close observation and considerable nursing care when admitted to the ward; the bed chosen should be in a position where this care can be readily available, whereas the patient who is admitted for diagnostic tests may prefer to have a bed in a quieter part of the ward, preferably with easy access to the dayroom, toilets and bathroom. This patient will prefer the company of more convalescent patients rather than being surrounded by the very ill, and the nurse should see that the patient is introduced to his neighbours, is shown the layout of the ward and knows when he may use the dayroom facilities for watching television or other such occupation. For the patient who is not feeling ill, time may seem to drag, and so it is important that some diversional therapy is introduced in the form of library books, the radio and visits from family and friends.

When the patient is admitted the nurse should check that all necessary details of the social history have been obtained, either by enquiry of the patient himself, or noting that the ward clerk has spoken to the patient and found out the relevant information regarding his address, next-of-kin and how to contact them should the need arise; also the name and address of the patient's general practitioner.

A full history will be taken by the doctor and a general examination carried out. As a result of this the doctor may arrange for several tests and investigations to be undertaken; it is the nurse's responsibility to see that the patient understands when these will be done, and to ensure that the patient is ready, suitably dressed, with notes and X-rays available for when he is collected to be taken to the special department for the various procedures.

Many patients prior to admission to hospital may have been receiving treatment from their own doctor for several weeks or months, and it is likely that they will bring their medicines into hospital with them; the nurse should tactfully acquire all such drugs and return them to the pharmacy, making sure the patient realizes that the doctor will prescribe drugs that are required and that they will be administered by the nursing staff. This is not only a safeguard for all patients and ward staff, but also allows the nurse to assess the effect of drugs given to the patient knowing the exact time and dose of all medicines administered.

NURSING OBSERVATIONS

An aid to diagnosis or progress can be provided by the accurate observations and records made by the nurse following admission of the patient. Such observations will include the temperature, pulse and respiratory rates, blood pressure, fluid intake and urinary output. Depending on the condition of the patient and the reason for admission, the temperature, pulse, respiration rates and blood pressure may only be recorded once daily. Gastrointestinal conditions often cause the patient to lose weight and therefore the weight may be recorded two or three times a week according to the wishes of the doctor. The patient may vomit, and the nurse should measure and observe the constituents of the vomit and record the time at which it occurred. She may also be asked to save a specimen. Alteration in bowel habits is a common feature of gastrointestinal conditions; the nurse should keep an accurate record of the number of bowel actions each day, and if the patient has diarrhoea a specimen of stool may be sent to the pathology department for culture and sensitivity. The patient may be concerned regarding constipation and this should be reported to the doctor, who may order an alteration to the diet or prescribe an aperient. The nurse should take note of the dietary habits of the patient, in particular observing what foods are avoided and how much is eaten. Many people with gastrointestinal upsets become fastidious about food and do not always appreciate that they can tolerate a normal diet, though they possibly suffer fewer symptoms if smaller and more frequent meals are taken. Observations should be made with regard to the type, time of occurrence and amount of pain that the patient experiences, and the nurse should note if this is relieved by food, medicines or activity, or whether these tend to increase the discomfort.

INVESTIGATIONS

Certain investigations are likely to be made whilst the patient is in hospital. Some are done routinely, such as the blood group, haemoglobin level, white and red cell counts and tests on the urine for protein, glucose, blood, bile and ketones. If these are found to be normal they will probably not be repeated, but if the haemoglobin level is found to be reduced from the normal (the average for an adult is 14·6 g/100 ml) this may require treatment and then further estimations will be made at intervals to note the effect of treatment. It is likely that some radiological investigations will be carried out, in particular a plain X-ray of the chest and abdomen. Some investigations will require the use of a radio-opaque substance such as barium, and the necessary preparation of the patient will be undertaken by the nurse; this will certainly include ensuring that the patient has not been given anything by mouth for the appropriate time prior to the investigation, and may necessitate giving a colonic washout prior to a barium enema. Certain procedures may require the patient to be given a local or general anaesthetic and the investigation is carried out in the operating theatre, the nurse having observed all the special aspects of nursing care relating to the patient undergoing anaesthesia. Such investigations include oesophagoscopy and gastroscopy, often with biopsy of the mucosa, and on completion the nurse must observe that the patient has a clear airway and ensure that nothing is given by mouth until the swallowing and cough reflexes have returned. For full details of all investigations carried out on the gastrointestinal tract, together with the preparation and aftercare of the patient see Chapter 14.

In some instances a provisional diagnosis is made that can only be confirmed when a laparotomy is performed. The patient should be told what is contemplated and give his consent for the surgeon to proceed with any operation that is found to be necessary. The nurse will be given guidance as to the preoperative preparations that are necessary, bearing in mind the anticipated outcome of the laparotomy.

GENERAL CARE

The nurse should ensure that her patient is as clean and comfortable as can be made possible. For the patient who is up and about in the ward it is usual for him to take a daily bath or shower, and facilities should be readily available for hand-washing after visits to the toilet; he should be encouraged in this respect. Spread of infection from the gastrointestinal tract is a common route, and, for the patient who has recently undergone surgery, may present as a severe complication, one that can often be avoided with attention to the cleanliness of baths and toilets, the personal hygiene of all patients and ward staff and care with the changing and handling of soiled bed linen.

Mattresses should be protected by a waterproof cover, similarly all pillows which are likely to become soiled by. leakage from wounds, vomit or gastric aspiration. The patient who is confined to bed should be provided with a drawsheet and mackintosh so that frequent changes of linen can be made and the bed kept fresh and clean. For the patient who is up and dressed for the greater part of the day a drawsheet is not necessary. A backrest or sufficient pillows should be used to enable the patient to rest comfortably in the upright position; these may be removed at night to enable him to sleep in a more familiar position. Bedclothes should be light in weight, and if necessary a bedcradle used. Many patients lose weight and in consequence are likely to become sore over bony prominences; hence great attention should be paid to the care of the skin, with frequent changes of position, application of barrier creams and the use of sheepskins, ripple mattresses and other appliances for relieving pressure.

In many gastrointestinal conditions the patient's mouth becomes dry and furred and develops an unpleasant taste. It is important that the nurse provides frequent mouthwashes and if the patient is unable to clean the mouth himself then a mouth tray should be provided and used frequently. The mouth is usually cleaned with a solution of bicarbonate of soda, followed by an antiseptic such as glycerine of thymol and the application of cream to the lips if they are dry and cracked. The nurse should see that dentures are cleaned twice a day or temporarily removed and kept in an antiseptic solution.

Following some operations on the digestive tract, leakage of intestinal juices occurs through the wound or drainage tube, the odour of which may be unpleasant and cause embarrassment to the patient. The nurse can assist here by changing or repacking the dressing frequently and by the discrete siting of a deodorant such as Airwick under, or by the bed.

The patient confined to bed should be given a daily bed bath and particular attention given to ensure that the flannel and towel used for the patient's face and upper part of the body does not come into contact with any secretions from operation sites. The use of disposable flannels and frequent changes of bath towels should be encouraged. Where there is a likelihood of spread of infection from the gastrointestinal tract the patient should be isolated or barrier nursed, care being exercised in the disposal of the contents of bedpans. If the patient is able to get up, one toilet should be allocated for the use of that person only and should be clearly labelled. In certain conditions, for example typhoid fever, it is necessary to disinfect stools by soaking them in a solution such as Sudol (1%) for one hour before emptying them into a bedpan sterilizer or disposable bedpan unit. Soiled bed linen should be sent for disinfection prior to laundering. The introduction of disposable crockery and cutlery has removed the necessity for keeping such equipment solely for that patient and disinfecting it after use.

DIET

For the majority of conditions affecting the digestive tract there is little need to alter the diet from a normal well balanced one of suitable proportions of protein foods, carbohydrate and fats, together with mineral salts, vitamins and water. A normal diet should contain foods which provide roughage; this will stimulate normal peristalsis in the gut and encourage regular defaecation. Foodstuffs which have a large roughage content are likely to provide a large food residue which is the form in which food reaches the large intestine. It is this residue which may require reduction in certain conditions such as regional ileitis, colitis, carcinoma and diverticulitis. Foods which contain roughage include green vegetables such as spinach and cabbage, onions, tomatoes, fruits including apples, pears, grapes, figs and prunes. Some of these foods should be included in the diet together with adequate quantities of fluid when treating the patient with atonic constipation (*see* page 189).

For many conditions a bland diet is ordered, that is, one that contains foods which do not cause chemical or mechanical irritation of the mucosa. Vegetables and fruit are taken in purée form. Foods should not be excessively sweet, sour, highly seasoned or served very hot or ice cold. Patients suffering from peptic ulceration may be advised to have a bland diet at the commencement of treatment, but as the ulcer heals there should be a gradual return to food served in the normal way. Many physicians adopt a liberal approach basing the diet on individual food tolerances and the response of the patient to treatment. Some patients find that tea, coffee and fried foods stimulate gastric secretions and increase the pain and therefore these are best avoided in the acute stage. A bland diet should contain a generous amount of milk and milk products, which help to counteract the acidity of the gastric contents and so reduce mucosal irritation and pain. Patients with peptic ulceration may be advised to take small, frequent and unhurried meals, thus avoiding long periods when only gastric juice is present in the stomach.

Certain conditions of the intestines give rise to the malabsorption syndrome in which the fat content of the diet is usually poorly absorbed. A reduction of fat in the diet reduces the large, bulky and greasy stools which are characteristic of these conditions. In some instances the gluten factor in the diet is responsible for the malabsorption syndrome. Reducing the intake of this protein which is found mainly in wheat (but also in rye and oats) and using soyabean flour or gluten-free wheat starch may promote a return to normal health.

Diseases of the liver or biliary apparatus often cause the patient to develop an intolerance to fatty foods. In the acute stages fat in the diet should be reduced and compensated for by giving adequate amount of protein and carbohydrate. The diet may contain bread, cereals, lean meat and poultry, not more than one egg a day and only if this is tolerated, a small quantity of butter, cooked vegetables and fruit. All fried foods and pastries should be avoided. When the acute stage has passed the patient may gradually introduce larger quantities of fat into the diet, up to a level which can be tolerated without discomfort.

METHODS OF FEEDING

Whichever method of feeding is employed the nurse should remember that in many instances the appetite will need to be tempted, and so the meal tray should look attractive, the food served appropriately hot or cold, offering a small amount at first with the choice of a further helping. Individual preferences, such as serving meals with or without gravy, should be noted. Before the tray is taken to the bedside the patient should be helped into a comfortable position having been given an opportunity to empty the bladder and wash the hands. Wherever possible meals should be taken seated at a table in the normal way, rather than in a cramped or unnatural position in bed. Mealtimes should be unhurried and the patient afforded a period of rest after eating.

Nasogastric feeds

For the patient who is too weak to eat or is unconscious, feeding by the nasogastric route is required.

Requirements:
Tray containing the feed at 38°C (100°F) in a measuring jug in a bowl of warm water; food thermometer; sterile polythene oesophageal catheter size 12 FG (6 EG); narrow funnel,

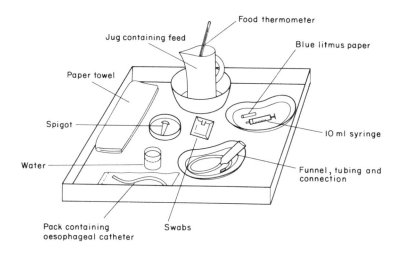

Food thermometer

Jug containing feed

Blue litmus paper

Paper towel

Spigot

10 ml syringe

Water

Funnel, tubing and connection

Pack containing oesophageal catheter

Swabs

Fig. 1. *Tray for nasogastric feed.*

tubing and tapered polythene connection 10 ml syringe; tray containing 2 gallipots, liquid paraffin or water, spigot and blue litmus paper; waterproof square and napkin; strapping; 50 ml warm water; mouth tray with spatula and gag; paper tissues; receiver.

Method

The patient is placed in a comfortable position and the nostrils cleaned if necessary. The waterproof square and napkin are placed in position. The catheter is lubricated and introduced along the floor of one nostril into the pharynx. The patient may assist the passage of the tube by swallowing. A length of tube comparable to the distance from the bridge of the nose to the xiphisternum is passed. The mouth is inspected using the spatula to note that the tube is not lying coiled in it. The tube is fastened to the cheek with strapping, a small quantity of fluid is aspirated through the tube and observed to turn blue litmus paper red. When the nurse is satisfied that the end of the tube is in the stomach the feed can be given. Twenty-five ml of water is poured into the funnel and allowed to run through the tubing to the end of the connection to expel air before attaching to the oesophageal tube. Provided the entry of the water is uneventful, the feed may be given, this should be run in slowly and on completion the remaining 25 ml of water is given to clean the tube. The apparatus is disconnected at the connection and the spigot inserted. The patient's mouth is cleaned and the details of the feed entered on the treatment chart. If the tube is to be withdrawn, it is pinched to avoid leakage of fluid into the larynx as it is removed. Feeds can be given at intervals through the tube which should be removed, cleaned and resterilized every twenty-four hours.

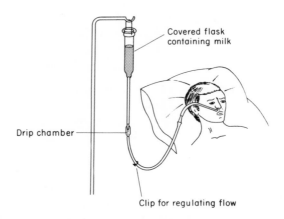

Covered flask
containing milk

Drip chamber

Clip for regulating flow

Fig. 2. *Continuous milk infusion.*

Milk feeds may be given as a continuous ('drip') method in some cases of peptic ulceration. Milk is allowed to drip slowly into the stomach from a reservoir, as much as two or three litres a day being given. The patient may be allowed to continue with normal oral feeds as well. The oesophageal tube is passed and checked to be in the stomach as for the nasogastric feed. The reservoir is filled with a measured amount of milk which is allowed to run through the two lengths of tubing and drip connection to the end of the tapered connection before the tube is clipped off. The apparatus is then connected to the oesophageal tube and the clip adjusted to allow a flow of about forty drops a minute. The reservoir must be covered and refilled when necessary with a measured amount of milk, and the details recorded.

Gastrostomy feeds

A gastrostomy is a permanent opening into the stomach through the abdominal wall, a catheter being sutured in place. This method of feeding may be used for patients with obstruction to the oesophagus usually resulting from a new growth. The catheter remains closed with a spigot. The nurse must endeavour to make the tray with the feed look attractive, and the patient may be permitted to suck a piece of fruit or any other food they fancy and spit it out again whilst the feed is being given in order to stimulate the secretion of gastric juice and to create an illusion of eating a meal.

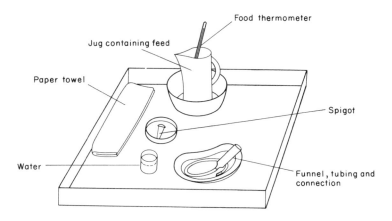

Fig. 3. *Tray for gastrostomy.*

Requirements:

Tray containing a small funnel; short length of tubing 20–25 cm and tapered polythene connection in a receiver; feed at 38°C (100°F) in a measuring jug in a bowl of warm water; food thermometer; 50 ml warm water; waterproof square and napkin.

Method

The patient is made comfortable, usually sitting upright, the waterproof square and napkin are place in position and the spigot is removed. After 25 ml of water has been poured into the funnel and allowed to pass through the tubing to the end of the tapered connection in order to expel air, the apparatus is connected to the gastrostomy tube and the water allowed to enter the stomach. It should be noted that the feed is given first, followed by any medicines and finally the remaining water to clean the tube. The feed should be given slowly: the flow is regulated by holding the funnel at about the level of the incision. On finishing the feed, the tubing is disconnected and the spigot introduced. Care should be taken to see that no gastric contents leak onto the skin where excoriation may occur and that the area around the gastrostomy tube is cleaned daily and the strapping renewed. Many patients return home with a gastrostomy tube in place, and so should be given opportunity whilst in the ward to help give their feed in order that confidence is gained before discharge from hospital.

Rectal infusion

Continuous rectal infusion may be used to supply fluid to a dehydrated patient often in the immediate post-operative period, although it is usual to maintain the fluid and electrolyte balance by the intravenous route.

Requirements:

Tray containing a reservoir; 2 lengths of tubing separated by a drip connection; a clip on the lower piece of tubing and a tapered polythene connection; catheter size 14 FG (6 EG);

jug of solution, usually tap water at 38°C (100°F); lotion thermometer; gallipot; lubricant; gauze squares and strapping; waterproof square and towel.

Method

The patient is placed in the left lateral position and the waterproof square and towel arranged under the buttocks. The catheter is lubricated and inserted into the rectum for a distance of 15 cm. The water is poured into the reservoir and allowed to pass through the tubing to the end of the tapered connection to expel air before the tube is clipped off. The apparatus is then attached to the rectal catheter and the clip adjusted to allow a flow of forty drops a minute and the tubing secured with strapping. The patient is then made comfortable. At intervals the reservoir will require refilling with a measured amount of fluid, and the patient observed to note that the fluid is being retained. If the patient feels distended or leakage of fluid occurs, the rate of flow should be reduced or temporarily suspended. Warm fluid is used when the infusion is set up but replenishments need only be at room temperature. An accurate record of the amount given should be kept.

NURSING PROCEDURES

Gastric aspiration

This procedure may be carried out for a variety of reasons which include diagnostic tests, immediately prior to surgery on the stomach and intestine and to relieve nausea and avoid vomiting both before and after operation.

Requirements:

Tray containing a Ryle's tube or polythene; oesophageal tube size 18 FG (10 EG) in a receiver; 2 gallipots; blue litmus paper; liquid paraffin; 50 ml syringe; measuring jug (500 ml); strapping; spigot; mouthwash; paper tissues;

vomit bowl; waterproof square and towel; container for dentures if required.

Method
The patient is placed in a comfortable position usually sitting upright, the waterproof square and towel are placed in position and dentures removed if present. The tube is lubricated and passed along the floor of one nostril to the pharynx. The patient may assist the passage of the tube by swallowing and when the tube is passed as far as the second mark the tip should be in the stomach. Then the mouth is checked to see that it does not contain a coiled tube, the syringe is attached and stomach contents withdrawn and the reaction to blue litmus paper noted. The tube is attached to the cheek with strapping and the spigot introduced. At intervals the stomach contents are aspirated, measured and recorded, the frequency being determined by the amount of aspirate and the need to prevent the patient feeling nauseated. Occasionally gastric aspiration is undertaken continuously; in this instance low power suction such as provided by a Roberts' sucker is used to create a vacuum in the drainage jar connected to the Ryle's tube.

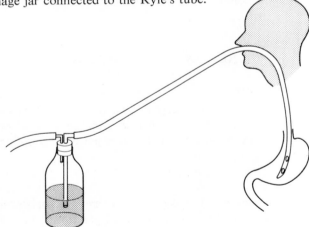

Fig. 4. *Continuous gastric aspiration.*

Intestinal aspiration

Aspiration of the intestine is usually carried out in cases of obstruction and may be undertaken by the use of a Miller Abbott tube. This is about 180 cm in length and consists of a double lumen, one to allow continuous suction and the other ending in a bag that can be inflated with air to aid peristalsis. The metal fitting at the end of the tube has two outlets marked 'filling' and 'suction'.

Requirements:
    As for gastric aspiration but using a Miller Abbott tube.

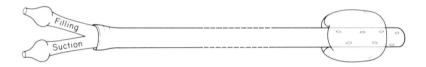

Fig. 5. *Miller Abbott type tube.*

Method
The nose may be sprayed with cocaine before the tube is passed as the end tends to be rather large and therefore uncomfortable for the patient. The tube is passed as far as the stomach, and the end attached loosely to the patient in order that it may travel further along the gut in the next few hours. Passage of the tube may be assisted by the patient lying on his right side for an hour or two. The balloon is inflated with air or water and the lumen closed by tying with thread. The tube is usually connected to apparatus for continuous suction as in gastric aspiration. When the tube has passed on into the intestine it must be left to continue on its way and when the tip appears at the anus the upper end is removed and the whole tube allowed to travel through. If the tube fails to pass into the duodenum it can be used for gastric aspiration and removed from the nose when no longer required.

Washouts

The stomach, colon and rectum may be irrigated in order to remove their contents, usually as a preparation before operation, although stomach washouts are used extensively in cases of non-corrosive poisoning. Warm water at 38°C (100°F) is used, and sometimes normal saline for a rectal washout: it is important that the temperature of the fluid is checked. These are socially clean procedures and therefore equipment need not be sterile. A known amount of fluid must be used as it is necessary for all of it to be recovered.

Stomach washout

This is used for cases of non-corrosive poisoning and as a preparation prior to operation on the stomach where stenosis has occurred. It is *not* a routine for all gastric surgery.

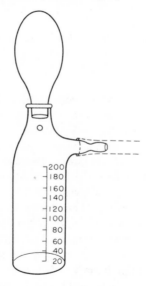

Fig. 6. *Senoran's evacuator.*

Requirements:
Trolley containing a funnel, tubing, clip and straight connection in a receiver; polythene oesophageal tube size 26–30 FG (15–18 EG); lotion thermometer; lotion in 3 litre jug at 38°C (100°F); water or normal saline; empty litre jug; Senoran's evacuator if required; jar for specimen of stomach contents; tray containing 2 gallipots and lubricant; waterproof square and towel; paper tissues; vomit bowl; mouthwash; bucket and floor rug; mouth gag and spatula for unconscious patient.

Method
If the patient is conscious and cooperative he should be sat upright and the procedure explained to him. The floor rug is spread beside the bed and the bucket placed on it. The waterproof square and towel are placed in position. The litre jug is filled from the large jug and the temperature of the water checked and the tube lubricated and introduced into the patient's mouth. The patient is encouraged to cooperate by swallowing when told to do so by the nurse and is asked not to bite on the tube but simply to close the lips over it. Time must be allowed for the patient to breathe quietly between swallowing, the nurse controlling the patient whilst this unpleasant procedure is taking place. When the tube is in the stomach it must be checked either by aspirating some of the stomach contents by using the Senoran's evacuator or by placing the end of the tube under water and noting whether bubbling occurs; bubbles which coincide with the respiratory rate indicate that the tube is in the trachea. To use the Senoran's evacuator it must be attached to the stomach tube, the bulb squeezed with one hand, and the hole covered by the thumb of the other hand. When the bulb is released the stomach contents flow into the flask; when the thumb is removed the flow ceases. The clip is attached and the funnel and tubing filled with solution and attached to the stomach tube. The tube is released and about 300 ml of fluid allowed to run in. Just before the funnel empties it is lowered to allow fluid rise in the funnel and is then inverted over the bucket and the fluid siphoned back. This is repeated until the returning fluid is clear. The

tube is then pinched and withdrawn and the patient given a mouth-wash.

The unconscious patient should be laid prone with the head turned to one side and the mouth opened with a gag. Some hospitals insist that a doctor passes a cuffed endotracheal tube before an unconscious patient is given a stomach washout.

Colonic washout

This procedure is used prior to some operations and investigations on the large intestine and where obstruction has occurred, often due to carcinoma. A large size catheter is used and the fluid siphoned back. If correctly carried out the procedure should empty the whole of the large intestine.

Requirements:

Trolley containing a funnel, tubing and tapered connection in a receiver; rectal tube or catheter size 30 FG (18 EG); water proof square and towel; floor rug and bucket; warm water at 38°C (100°F) up to 10 litres in amount; lubricant and swabs; litre jug; lotion thermometer.

Method

The patient is placed comfortably in the left lateral position and covered with a blanket with the waterproof and towel arranged under the buttocks. The floor rug is spread beside the bed and the bucket placed on it. Water is poured into the litre jug and the temperature checked. The catheter is lubricated and inserted as far as possible into the rectum. Water is poured into the funnel and allowed to flow through the tubing to the end of the tapered connection to expel air before attaching it to the rectal catheter. The fluid is run gently into the rectum and just before it all leaves the funnel, the funnel is lowered to allow fluid to flow back into it. It is then inverted over the bucket and the fluid siphoned back. The procedure is repeated until the returning fluid is clear; this may take as much as 10 litres of water to achieve. It is important that a known quantity of fluid is used and that it is all recovered.

Rectal washout

This is the introduction of not more than 500 – 1000 ml of warm water or normal saline into the rectum and then siphoning it back. It is used as a final preparation before operations on the rectum, where it is necessary to remove mucus or blood.

Requirements:
As for colonic washout except that a smaller rectal catheter is used and only 500 – 1000 ml of solution.

Method
As for colonic washout, allowing the introduction of 120 ml of solution before siphoning it back. It is very important that all the fluid introduced is returned; it should be measured and recorded.

Colostomy washout

This procedure may need to be carried out following operations on the large intestine usually for carcinoma. It is strictly speaking not a washout but an enema given through the colostomy. Details of the procedure are given in Chapter 10.

PREPARATION FOR SURGERY

Wherever possible adequate time must be available for both the physical and mental preparation of the patient about to undergo an operation. This usually means that the patient is admitted to the ward about forty-eight hours prior to surgery; longer if certain investigations need to be carried out or pre-operative procedures such as daily colonic washout before some operations on the intestine. The patient must have confidence in the surgeon and nurses who will care for him. An explanation of the operation should be given in terms which he can understand, questions answered and an outline of the pre- and post-operative regimen described so that the patient is cooperative and realizes the necessity for certain procedures or treatments that he experiences. The patient who has had a chronic blood loss from a peptic ulcer over a period of time may be found to be anaemic when blood investigations are carried out on admission; operation may be delayed until a blood transfusion has been given and the general health improved. Some operations require extensive preoperative preparation of the gut, and these measures are dealt with in more detail where the condition is discussed in the appropriate chapter. In general, the stomach needs to be empty, either by withholding food for six hours and fluid for four hours prior to operation or by passing a Ryle's tube and aspirating the gastric contents. Similarly the bowel should be empty, and it is usual to give an enema or suppositories the day before operation to facilitate a bowel action. Local preparation of the skin over the operation site amounts to shaving the area carefully, using soap and water in preference to a dry shave, allowing the patient to take a bath if possible and ensuring that the skin and umbilicus are clean. The patient should be encouraged to sleep well the night before operation and a mild hypnotic may be given to achieve this and allay anxiety.

Immediately prior to operation the patient should be dressed in an operation gown and socks, the bladder should be emptied, an identity band bearing the patient's name and registry number is put on (if this has not been done on admission), all prostheses removed, long hair tied back, jewellery, lipstick and nail varnish removed. Some women prefer to retain their wedding ring and this should be covered with zinc oxide plaster. All jewellery removed must be clearly labelled and locked in a cupboard. The nurse is responsible for checking that the patient has signed the consent for anaesthesia and operation form, that the premedication is given when directed by the anaesthetist and the patient made comfortable in bed and able to rest quietly. The details of drugs given, the time and amount of urine passed together with the results of testing a recent specimen of urine are entered on the consent for operation form and left ready with the patient's notes, X-rays and pathology reports. The theatre technician who collects the patient should bring a written request, by which the nurse can check that the correct patient is taken to theatre; the nurse accompanying the patient and remaining with him in the anaesthetic room until either the patient is unconscious or she is relieved by the theatre nurse.

Once the patient has gone to theatre the bed should be stripped and remade with clean sheets, drawsheet and mackintosh, sufficient pillows are placed near the bed and the locker cleared and prepared. On the locker should be placed a vomit bowl and paper tissues, receiver for the artificial airway, anaesthetic instruments (those accompanying the patient to and from theatre may be used), sphygmomanometer, stethoscope and thermometer. An infusion stand, suction apparatus and sterile tubing may be required. A treatment chart should be prepared.

POST-OPERATIVE CARE

The nurse will go to theatre to collect her patient and will be given a verbal message about the operation that has taken place, the condition of the patient and any instructions concerning the immediate nursing care. The colour and pulse rate of the patient should be satisfactory before the nurse returns with the patient to the ward or recovery unit. The nurse walks alongside the trolley at the head of the patient, maintaining the head on one side and the jaw held forward to support the tongue. The bed should be screened whilst the patient is settled comfortably usually on one side. The dressing should be inspected before the top bedclothes are put over the patient. The container of intravenous fluid is placed on the infusion stand and the intragastric tube connected to the suction apparatus if indicated. The patient's temperature (axillary) pulse and respiratory rates and blood pressure are taken and recorded. It is essential that a nurse remains with the patient until consciousness is regained; in so doing the patient will reject the artificial airway which should be placed in the receiver. One or more pillows may then be put under the patient's head. It is customary to get the patient into a recumbent position as soon as possible following a return to consciousness.

Observation of the patient's colour, the temperature, pulse and respiratory rates will be made and recorded at intervals depending on the general condition. It should be noted when the patient passes urine and an accurate fluid intake and urina y output kept. Pain will be experienced and the nurse should see that the appropriate analgesic is given and note the effect that this has on the discomfort. A Ryle's tube will need to be aspirated. The frequency of this is determined by the amount of aspirate and by whether or not the patient feels nauseated. The tube is removed when it is no longer necessary. The dressing should be inspected, and if leakage from the wound is excessive then repacking or renewal of the dressing is indicated. Mouthwashes should be given frequently, the patient bedbathed and given clean nightclothes. Following some operations on the gut fluids by mouth are withheld until bowel sounds return usually about 24–36 hours post-operatively; small quantities of fluid should be given at first when directed by the doctor. Once fluids by mouth are tolerated a light diet may be commenced progressing to a full diet in a few days if all is well.

Movement in bed and ambulation is encouraged for the majority of patients. When the patient first starts to walk the abdominal wound may be uncomfortable and the nurse should encourage an upright posture. Deep breathing exercises will be taught and the patient should be shown how to support the sides of the wound whilst coughing. Care of the wound varies according to the operation performed, but the stab drainage tube (if present) may be removed or shortened after about forty-eight hours, and is likely not to be required after about the fourth post-operative day. Abdominal sutures are removed between the seventh and twelfth days. Up till the time of removal of the sutures the wound may be covered with an adhesive dressing which does not require changing. Provided the patient feels well, a daily bath or shower may be taken or else a bed bath is given.

At all times in the post-operative period the nurse must be aware of possible complications that can arise, reporting immediately if the patient has a pyrexia, complains of pain in the wound, chest or calves or has a haemorrhage. Other complications which might occur are vomiting, urinary retention and subsequent infection, and abdominal distension due to flatus collecting in the inactive gut. The latter is common on about the second and third post-operative days after surgery on the gut and may be relieved by early mobilization, administering peppermint water or by passing a flatus tube. The flatus tube is lubricated and introduced about 15 cm into the rectum, the patient having been placed comfortably in the lateral position. The flatus tube is connected to a length of tubing, the end of which lies in a bowl of water. The tube is left in place for about ten minutes when relief will be experienced. The use of suppositories or an enema on about the fourth day may help to overcome constipation and gentle aperients may need to be given for the next few days until normal bowel habits are regained.

DISCHARGE FROM HOSPITAL AND AFTERCARE

The patient will look forward with eagerness to his discharge from hospital; he expects to return home feeling well and confident that he will remain so. For many, discharge from hospital means a return home to the welcome of family and friends, and after a period of convalescence, a return to work. Just as the patient is anxious to return to his familiar surroundings so are the family eager to receive and help him adjust to a normal home life again. For others, leaving hospital means separation from people and the newly made friends to return perhaps to living on one's own with little contact with the outside world; for this person who may not feel really fit, painful symptoms may become exaggerated and slow progress made towards a full recovery unless definite steps are taken to see that this patient is once again integrated into the community.

Often when the patient enters hospital some guidance can be given as to when to expect to be discharged, but where possible several days' notice should be given to both the patient and his relatives. This will make the progression from hospital to home smoother if the family have had sufficient time to prepare for the return of the patient. Before discharge from hospital the patient should be examined by the doctor; this will give the latter an opportunity to discuss any specific measures with regard to increase of activities or future plans regarding treatment, and also to answer questions. Any drugs or medical supplies that the patient will need at home should be prescribed by the doctor well in advance of the patient leaving hospital, to give the nursing staff time to acquire these from the appropriate department.

Some patients will return home with a new colostomy or gastrostomy tube in place. It is essential that the patient has had ample opportunity whilst in the ward to acquire the skill of caring for this and knows exactly how to manage the dressing or give the feeds. The patient will require dressings and sufficient should be supplied to last for several days so the patient does not need to visit his general practitioner for a prescription immediately on leaving hospital. Information should be given as to how to renew supplies of equipment and what to do if an emergency arises. Some patients may benefit from being put in touch with certain organizations such as the Ileostomy Association where they know they will receive helpful advice.

Skilled nursing care may still be required at home by some patients and the nurse should see that adequate arrangements are made before the patient leaves hospital. Many patients may already know their district nurse but for some this will be a new experience and they should know her name, where to contact her and when she is likely to make a first visit to them. The nurse, on the other hand, should be given all the relevant details concerning the patient's diagnosis, treatment and aftercare required, together with some information about the mobility of the patient and who is at home to help look after them. If these arrangements are made by telephone, confirmation should be given in writing at the earliest opportunity. In some areas of the country arrangements for home nursing are made directly between the ward sister and the district nurse; in others this may go to the Divisional Nursing Officer with responsibility for the community or to the general practitioner. Similarly, the general practitioner should be given the same details as soon as possible, for if the patient is unwell when he returns home it is the doctor who will be called and who needs to know what has happened during the patient's stay in hospital.

Other services may be required by the patient after returning home. These include ambulance or other transport to enable the patient to return to hospital for treatment or attend a follow-up clinic, a home help and possibly meals-on-wheels. Arrangements for these should be made well in advance of the patient being discharged from hospital so that they know exactly what has been planned. All patients will be seen in a follow-up clinic within a few days or weeks of leaving hospital; an appointment should be made and the patient know where and when he is expected to attend.

The nurse should strive from the outset to make the patient's stay in hospital as comfortable and free from pain and anxiety as possible and help him to become independent again and ready to return home, the transition from one stage to the next being made as smooth as possible with foresight and careful planning.

CHAPTER 2

The Mouth

The structures which form the boundaries of the mouth develop around the opening of the foregut early in intrauterine life. The mouth is separated from the nasal cavity above by the palate, and below, the floor of the mouth is formed mainly by the tongue and its supporting musculature which is inserted into the hyoid bone. The cheeks, or side walls of the mouth, develop from an ingrowing of the maxillary process on each side. Development of the palate and related structures is a very complicated process and it is no wonder that failure of fusion to a greater or lesser extent not infrequently occurs, giving rise to the relatively common congenital anomalies of cleft lip and palate.

Development of the face and palate

The face develops from five bony processes:

(a) The frontonasal process which projects downwards from the cranium and will form the nose, nasal septum and premaxilla (a V-shaped central anterior portion of the upper jaw which bears the four incisor teeth).

(b) Two maxillary processes, one on each side which fuse with each other in the midline and above with the frontonasal process to form the checks, upper lip, upper jaw and the palate (except the premaxilla).

(c) Two mandibular processes, one from each side which fuse in
the midline to form the lower jaw.

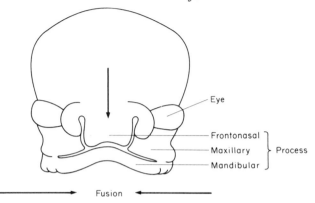

Fig. 7. *Development of the face (arrows indicate direction of growth).*

The palate separates the nasal and buccal cavities and is formed
of two parts, the vault-shaped hard palate which merges posteriorly
with the soft palate; this latter hangs between the naso- and oro-
pharynx. Centrally, from its posterior edge hangs the uvula and
laterally it merges into the anterior and posterior pillars of the fauces,
between which are to be found the tonsils. During development the
roof of the mouth becomes more arched, and with growth of the
neck and mandible the tongue sinks below the level of the primitive
palate thus allowing the palatal processes to grow in the horizontal
plane to fuse in the midline to form the palate. At the same time the
lower free edge of the nasal septum grows downwards to complete
the fusion (like an inverted T⊥) and thus form the boundaries of the
nasal fossae and mouth. Ossification occurs later.

The tonsils are composed of lymphoid tissue covered over by
squamous epithelium pitted by up to twenty crypts. The tonsillar
branch of the facial artery supplies the tonsil, and the lymphatic
drainage is to the nodes alongside the internal jugular vein at the
angle of the jaw. Progressive atrophy of the tonsil takes place from
late puberty.

Development of the floor of the mouth and tongue

The mylohyoid muscles form a sling which supports the tongue as they pass from the sides of the mandible to be inserted into the hyoid bone. Above the muscle are the sublingual salivary glands and below, the submandibular glands with their associated lymph nodes.

The tongue bears a V-shaped groove on its dorsal surface which divides it into a buccal and a pharyngeal portion. A shallow groove indicates the median vertical fibrous septum, on either side of which are situated the intrinsic and extrinsic muscles of the tongue; the former alter the shape of the tongue and the latter move the tongue as a whole. These muscles pass from the mandible, hyoid bone and soft palate to insert into the tongue. On either side of the frenulum (a fold of mucous membrane connecting the anterior part of the tongue to the floor of the mouth) on the under aspect of the tongue can be seen the lingual veins supported by thin mucosa, more deeply will be found the lingual artery and nerve. The dorsal surface is of thick squamous epithelium which contains papillae over its anterior two-thirds, the posterior part bearing lymphoid tissue which with the tonsils and adenoids completes a lymphoid ring. The lymph drains to three groups of lymph nodes situated under the chin and mandible, and the deep cervical chain.

There are three types of papillae which bear special receptors, the taste buds: fungiform papillae are present on the tip and edges of

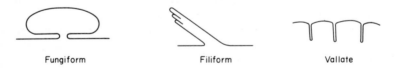

Fungiform   Filiform   Vallate

Fig. 8. *Tongue papillae.*

the tongue being bright red and mushroom-shaped; filiform papillae are long and slender and are also found along the tongue edge and the anterior aspect. The superficial cell layers covering these are continuously shed and if this process becomes arrested then a furred tongue results. Vallate papillae are rather like squat towers situated at the back of the tongue and are the chief ones to bear taste buds. The taste buds are a collection of specialized cells opening onto the surface by the gustatory pore, and from the base of the bud nerve fibres pass to the facial and glossopharyngeal nerves which relay taste sensations to the cerebral cortex. The lingual branch of the

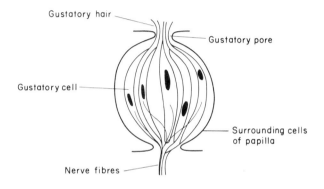

Fig. 9. *Taste bud.*

trigeminal nerve is responsible for relaying impulses of pain, temperature and touch, all of which assist in the interpretation of taste. Only substances in solution can be tasted, and one of the functions of saliva is to facilitate this. The four primary taste sensations are sweet, sour, salt and bitter; sour and salt are appreciated on the sides of the tongue; salt and sweet on the tip and bitter towards the back of the tongue.

Salivary glands

The salivary glands are three pairs of glands formed as solid outgrowths of the buccal epithelium, and during development their ducts become elongated. The largest of these glands are the parotid glands situated wedged between the sternomastoid muscle and the mandible. The investing fascia of this gland is thicker both in front and below; this forms the only separation from the adjacent submandibular gland.

The parotid glands

These glands are crossed by the facial nerve, the posterior facial vein and the external carotid artery prior to its dividing into temporal and maxillary branches. The facial nerve branches either just before or just after entering the parotid gland to form the upper temporal, zygomatic and buccal branches, and the lower mandibular and cervical branches. The duct (of Stensen) leads from the anterior part of the gland, passes over the masseter muscle and opens opposite the second upper molar tooth; it is 5 cm in length.

The submandibular glands

These glands are situated close to the mylohyoid muscles in the floor of the mouth and pour their secretion along Wharton's duct which opens in the mouth at the side of the frenulum. The cervical branch of the facial nerve crosses the gland, and the facial artery is associated with the posterior and superior aspects of this gland.

The sublingual glands

These glands lie on the lateral aspects of Wharton's duct and open into the floor of the mouth by upwards of twenty small ducts. The lingual nerves cross the gland as they pass to the tongue. Both sympathetic and parasympathetic nerve fibres supply the salivary glands, and secretion of saliva is largely the result of reflex activity stimulated by the presence of food in the mouth coming into contact with the taste buds, teeth and oral mucosa. About $1-1\cdot5$ l of saliva are produced daily, by far the greater proportion coming from the submandibular glands. Saliva is a viscous, colourless fluid with a pH of $6\cdot2-7\cdot4$, containing only about $0\cdot5\%$ solids in the form of organic matter, principally mucin and the enzyme α amylase (ptyalin); this latter is contained in the zymogen granules in the serous cells.

Mastication has the effect of bringing saliva into close contact with the particles of food thus allowing the enzyme to start the breakdown of cooked starch to maltose. Saliva also provides a solvent necessary for the preparation of food for swallowing. It also helps in speaking and has a cleansing effect on the mouth and teeth by the bactericidal action of the constituent lysozyme. Saliva also has a buffering action brought about by the bicarbonate, phosphate and mucin which it contains. Some contribution towards the body's regulation of water balance is made by the suppression of secretion when there is a need to conserve water; this results in a dry mouth and sensation of thirst.

Development of the lips, cheeks and gums

The mandibular processes as they grow in towards the midline develop a groove thus separating areas of tissue which in turn will differentiate into the lower lip and gum. The lateral upper parts of the lip and gum are formed in a similar way from the maxillary processes, and the central portion develops from a downgrowth of the frontonasal process which ultimately fuses on either side. Progressive fusion of the upper and lower lips at the angle of the mouth gives rise to the formation of the cheeks.

Deglutition (swallowing)

The process of swallowing can be best considered as comprising three stages: buccal, pharyngeal and oesophageal; only the first is under voluntary control. The bolus of food is pushed backwards by the action of the tongue pressing against the hard palate. At the same time the soft palate rises to close off the nasopharynx and respiration is inhibited. As the food reaches the back of the tongue the larynx rises causing the bolus to press against the epiglottis which is forming a protective hood over the entrance to the larynx. At this stage the process becomes involuntary and the bolus is steered into the oesophagus and is conveyed down partly by gravity and partly by peristalsis. Once the food has passed safely into the oesophagus the larynx descends, the tongue passes forwards, the epiglottis recoils to regain its former position and respiration continues.

CONGENITAL ANOMALIES

Cleft lip and palate

The main anomalies found are those relating to failure of fusion of the lip or palate or both. The combination of cleft palate and cleft lip is twice as common as cleft palate or cleft lip occurring alone, and of these the majority are to be found in male babies. Unilateral cleft of the palate or lips is more common than bilateral. Causes of this congenital anomaly may be attributed to heredity, or other factors such as rubella in early pregnancy, exposure to X-rays or possible steroid toxicity. It is not uncommon for a cleft palate or lip to be only one of a number of congenital abnormalities present.

The effect of a cleft lip is only minimal and should not give rise to major problems of feeding the baby, but will require repairing at a suitable age mainly for cosmetic reasons and also to ensure correct speech and development of the nose. However, as far as the parents are concerned, as the lip is readily visible, it causes them a great deal of distress and seems far more serious than the cleft palate; they will need a great deal of help and support at this time. On the other hand, the baby with a cleft palate poses a problem of feeding, and it is essential that the palate is repaired to enable speech and the correct positioning of the teeth to take place. Some babies may suffer from a slight hearing defect due to oedema of the lower part of the Eustachian tube resulting from persistent inflammation caused by regurgitation of food. Surgical repair of these anomalies is usually in the sphere of the surgeon who specializes in faciomaxillary work. The timing of the operation varies, but many would agree that the lip should be repaired when the baby is about three months old or weighs 6 kg (13·2 lb) and the palate at between twelve and eighteen months. Following repair of a cleft palate care will need to be taken regarding speech training and orthodontics. Prior to repair of the cleft palate the baby may be fed using a special teat which has an additional flange over the top of it which makes up for the deficiency in the palate and prevents regurgitation of the feed into the nostrils, or a specially constructed spoon with a lid and small outlet channel. Some mothers may prefer to breast feed their baby but may find this very difficult unless they have long nipples, in which case expressed

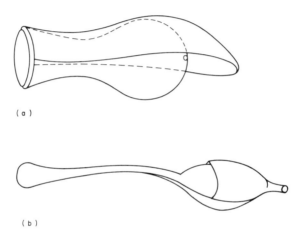

(a)

(b)

Fig. 10. (a) *Modified teat for feeding baby with cleft palate;* (b) *Modified teaspoon for feeding baby with cleft palate.*

breast milk may be given by either bottle or spoon. When solids are introduced into the diet they should be in a soft and easily swallowed form; they will need to be given slowly by spoon allowing the baby time to swallow and then breathe, or the food will readily pass into the nose obstructing the airway and cause the baby to panic. The baby should be sitting in an upright position whilst being fed.

Following operation it is important that some restraint is put on the baby's arms to prevent him touching the delicate suturing of the lip or the inside of mouth. Great care must be taken when feeding the baby not to cause damage with the spoon and the suture lines should be carefully cleaned at the conclusion of each feed using a solution of hydrogen peroxide (one part in eight parts water). Following repair of the palate a drink of water may be given to clean the mouth after giving a meal of a semisolid consistency. Until healing has taken place the baby should be discouraged from putting things into his mouth, but as an added precaution all toys should be of the soft variety. It is also important that no undue tension is put on the suture lines and so crying should be prevented even if this means a little extra attention and cuddling, and occasionally the administration of a sedative may be necessary. Sutures are usually of catgut and will therefore not require removal, but if silk has been used then these should be taken out on about the sixth postoperative day. Further minor plastic surgery may need to be undertaken when the child is three or four years old, mainly for cosmetic reasons.

Abnormalities of the jaw

These abnormalities rarely occur but may be associated with a cleft palate. Micronathia, or lack of development of the mandible may occur resulting in feeding problems and tongue swallowing, causing dyspnoea and cyanosis. Nursing care is devoted to maintaining a clear airway and overcoming the feeding difficulties until puberty is reached when bone grafting may be undertaken. Agnathia, or absence of the lower jaw may also occur.

Tongue tie

In some instances the baby may be born with a short frenulum which prevents the tongue from extending beyond the teeth; if this is only of a mild degree then it will probably right itself as the child grows, but just occasionally it is necessary to carry out a minor operation and divide the frenulum.

TRAUMA

Injuries to the mouth and jaw include lacerations of the mouth and tongue such as may happen to the epileptic during a fit, or those caused by a sudden blow or fall sufficient to break the stem of a pipe being smoked and drive the broken ends into the tongue. These injuries will require control of the bleeding and suturing of the laceration. Minor trauma may be caused by sharp edges on teeth or incorrectly fitting dentures.

Other traumatic conditions are usually of the more serious type and involve fractures and lacerations such as may be sustained in a road traffic accident where the casualty is flung through the windscreen of the vehicle. The repair of these injuries and the subsequent nursing care is more within the scope of the faciomaxillary surgeon and his team and for this reason has not been included in a book on gastroenterology.

INFLAMMATORY CONDITIONS

Inflammation in the mouth, or stomatitis, may be due to a number of causes of which probably the chief ones are those associated with the administration of certain drugs, blood diseases and a deficiency of vitamins in the diet.

Stomatitis due to chemotherapy

This may present as an occupational hazard to persons who handle large quantities of mercury, or as a complication of treatment with mercurial diuretics. In both cases removal of the source of the mercury should bring about improvement in the condition of the mouth; if not Dimercaprol (BAL) solution 50 mg in 1 ml is given by deep intramuscular injection; this has the effect of combining with the heavy metal to form a stable compound which is readily excreted by the kidneys. Lead may also cause stomatitis, either in those whose work involves handling lead or in young children who may continually suck toys or cot sides painted with a high lead content paint. In these days this latter cause should not occur as there is a wide variety of safe paints on the market. Diagnosis may be assisted by observing the presence of a blue line along the gums. As well as removing the source of the lead the patient should be treated for other signs of chronic lead poisoning, particular attention being paid to conditions of the renal tract and haemolytic anaemia. Sodium calciumedetate may be given intravenously in a $0\cdot5$–3% solution added to 250–500 ml of normal saline or dextrose saline adminstered over a period of one hour. Epileptic patients receiving phenytoin may find that in time overgrowth of the gums occurs leading to gingivitis in which case another anticonvulsant should be used. An allergic reaction to certain antibiotics may give rise to stomatitis; this may also be associated with alteration in the intestinal bacterial flora, resulting in a vitamin deficiency. Occasionally the condition occurs as a local allergic reaction to toothpaste or new dentures.

Stomatitis as a complication of blood diseases

Such conditions as agranulocytosis, leukaemia, pernicious anaemia, iron deficiency anaemia and thrombocytopenic purpura may result in stomatitis occurring with an associated fungus infection. Improvement in the condition of the mouth will usually be seen when the underlying cause responds to treatment. In the meantime, nystatin mouthwashes 100 000 units in 1 ml may be given at two hourly intervals, and analgesic lozenges containing amethocaine may be prescribed.

Stomatitis due to vitamin deficiency

Inflammation of the tongue (glossitis) may be the main feature of this form of stomatitis resulting from a nutritional dificiency of vitamins. Attention to the dietary needs of the patient should bring about improvement in the condition.

INFECTIVE CONDITIONS

Moniliasis

Probably the most common infection of the mouth that the nurse is likely to see is monilia (thrush) caused by the fungus *Candida albicans*, a condition which may occur at any age. It is characterized by white plaques which are firmly adhered to the mucosa. In babies, thrush may result from infection acquired during birth from the mother who has not received adequate treatment for this type of infection occurring in the vagina during pregnancy. Alteration in hormonal levels and changes in vaginal acidity occurring during pregnancy make thrush a common minor complication. Thrush may spread rapidly amongst newborn babies if communal feeding utensils are inadequately sterilized. In adults the condition may occur as a complication of certain gastrointestinal diseases, especially ulcerative colitis, and the lesions may extend from the mouth into the oesophagus. Alteration to the intestinal bacterial flora induced by the oral administration of some broad spectrum antibiotics may also predispose to the occurrence of this fungal infection. Diagnosis may be assisted by bacteriological examination of a small area of the lesion gently scraped from the plaque with a wooden spatula. The fact that the characteristic white plaques on the mucous membranes within the mouth are adherent and not easily removed, is one way in which the nurse may differentiate between thrush and milk curds seen in the baby's mouth immediately after a feed. At whatever age oral thrush occurs it causes soreness during eating and results in general ill health and failure to maintain or gain weight. Treatment is by improving nutrition and by giving additional vitamins of the B group, together with local application of nystatin tablets containing 500 000–1 million units six hourly for adults, or nystatin in honey 1 million units in 1 ml four times a day for babies. In either case if the fungal infection proves resistant to nystatin, the area may be painted with a 1% aqueous solution of gentian violet. Although for cosmetic reasons this latter treatment is rarely used it still remains a very effective form of therapy. In all cases strict attention to oral hygiene should be given, and possible spread of infection by contaminated cups, cutlery or, in the case of babies, feeding bottles and teats, should be prevented by adequate sterilization of all such equipment.

Gingivitis

Gingivitis (inflammation of the gums) may become a septic condition complicated by the increase in organisms present in the mouth resulting in pyorrhoea. Poor oral hygiene is often the cause, and attention to this should be given. The infected material from around the teeth is likely to be swallowed and on reaching the stomach may give rise to gastritis.

Syphilis

Syphilitic lesions occur in the mouth and may be present in any of the three stages. The chancre or primary lesion is found on the lip or tongue and contains many treponemes; in secondary syphilis ulceration of the mucosa giving rise to the characteristic 'snail track' lesions is also highly infectious. The gumma of tertiary syphilis may occur in the mouth and appear to mimic a carcinoma—it is not impossible that they may in time become one—but these lesions are not infective. Treatment of syphilis should be undertaken at the earliest possible opportunity by giving large doses of penicillin systemically.

Other infective conditions occurring in the mouth may result from virus infection, particularly those of herpes simplex and herpes zoster. In caring for patients with infections in the mouth the nurse should encourage frequent attention to oral hygiene by the use of mouthwashes especially after meals. When there is no longer infection present dental examination should be carried out and any carious teeth treated.

Salivary infections

Infection of the salivary glands may occur. This may be epidemic parotitis (mumps), a virus infection; a description of this condition does not come within the context of gastroenterology and the reader is referred to a textbook dealing with the communicable diseases. The condition of acute suppurative parotitis may result from ascending infection from the mouth, travelling through the ducts of the salivary glands; usually the organisms *Staphylococcus aureus* or *Streptococcus pyogenes* are responsible. This condition may occur as a complication of intestinal disease where pyrexia and dehydration are present. Treatment is effected by the administration of the appropriate antibiotic. Infection may also be associated with the presence of a calculus in the duct leading from a salivary gland, usually the submaxillary gland. The gland swells and causes pain whilst eating. Diagnosis is confirmed by X-ray and occasionally a sialogram (*see* page 285) may be necessary. Treatment consists of surgical removal of the calculus, together with the administration of an antibiotic.

Vincent's agina

Vincent's angina is an infective condition of the fauces in which they become covered by a yellowish/white slough. Two organisms are responsible; the bacillus fusiformis and Vincent's spirochaete. A virus may also be present. The condition can also affect the gums causing them to become red, swollen and have a tendency to bleed. Halitosis may occur. Systemic administration of penicillin is used to treat this condition.

NEOPLASTIC CONDITIONS

Neoplasms occurring in the mouth may be either benign or malignant; the former are of various types and their treatment comes mainly within the scope of the dental surgeon and will therefore not be considered here. The squamous cell carcinoma of the mouth is the most common of malignant tumours; this usually starts on the lower lip and spreads to the regional lymph nodes. In carcinoma of the tongue the anterior two-thirds is mainly affected, and treatment is usually by radiotherapy (implantation of radium needles), or surgery where the affected area of the tongue is excised (hemiglossectomy), or a combination of both methods of treatment. White plaques that are either smooth or raised may be present on the surface of the tongue and may be indicative of the condition of leukoplakia—this is a pre-malignant state which may respond to early treatment with the administration of vitamin B complex in large doses. Chronic iron deficiency anaemia with associated mucosal atrophy may predispose to dysphagia (Plummer–Vinson syndrome). This is a pre-malignant condition which occurs more frequently in women and which may lead to post-cricoid carcinoma. Malignant conditions occurring in the tonsils are mostly commonly the lymphosarcoma. In all of these conditions the patient is likely to experience dysphagia, the sensation of a lump in the throat, changes in the quality of the voice and sometimes pain in the ear.

Malignant tumours in the salivary glands are usually of the mixed variety and affect mainly the parotid glands. For this reason they may interfere with movements of the jaw and give rise to facial palsy and deafness. Diagnosis can be assisted by sialography which entails passing a cannula into Stensen's duct, introducing a radio-opaque substance such as lipiodol and then taking an X-ray. Treatment consists of radiotherapy, surgical excision or a combination of both.

NURSING CARE

In considering the abnormal conditions which can occur in the mouth it should be noted that certain features are common to many of them, of these perhaps fetor due to a bacterial stomatitis giving rise to halitosis is the most unpleasant. In caring for the sick the nurse should realize that the patient may be only too aware that to come into close proximity with him is distasteful to other members of the ward and the nursing team, and for this reason the patient may tend to isolate himself. By tactful encouragement and frequent provision of the necessary facilities for oral hygienic care the nurse can do a lot to help both the physical and psychological comfort of her patient. In the more advanced stages of carcinoma of the mouth the use of irrigations with hypochlorite or a strategically placed deodorant aerosol may prevent considerable embarrassment to the patient and make visiting time a more pleasurable experience for the relatives. Salivation may be increased in case of malignant tumours, and where there is difficulty in swallowing then excess saliva may continually dribble from the mouth. This is not only unpleasant for the patient but may lead to excoriation of the skin around the mouth and chin. The patient should be well supplied with soft paper tissues or small gauze squares for mopping the saliva and have a suitable receptacle at hand for their disposal, the nurse checking to see that this is changed frequently. Alteration in the quantity of saliva or the presence of a tumour in the mouth may present difficulties in articulation, and the patient may find he is not readily understood; this leads to frustration and annoyance on the part of the patient and sometimes impatience on the part of those dealing with him. Keeping the mouth moist may help with speech difficulties. The assistance of a speech therapist and above all a very tolerant attitude on the part of the nursing team may go some way towards helping a patient with this problem. The most natural and effective way is to increase the output from the salivary glands which may be achieved by chewing astringent foods such as fresh pineapple or lemon, although it must be remembered that if parotitis is present this will increase the pain.

When dysphagia is present consideration must be given to the patient's diet, as it is only too easy for the patient to have an insufficient calorie and fluid intake during the day if feeding is both painful and slow. Of necessity foodstuffs will need to be soft, but the nurse should see that meals are not only colourful and look attractive, but that the patient is unhurried and, if he prefers, is allowed to eat quietly on his own and not made to take his meals sitting at a table in company with more able people. The use of a liquidizer may be invaluable in maintaining a patient on a normal balanced diet, both from a nutritional content and the fact that the patient knows he is having the food that he has smelt and fancied. At the conclusion of the meal the mouth should be thoroughly cleaned, using a bicarbonate of soda solution (3 g/600 ml water) followed by a glycerine of thymol rinse. It is important for any patient with dysphagia who has a long term feeding problem to be weighed frequently, as this will give a clear indication as to whether the nutritional intake is adequate to maintain body weight.

Carious teeth may be a source of infection and halitosis, and dental examination should be carried out and any necessary treatment given. For the endentulous patient, consideration to their dentures (and possible encouragement to wear them) may improve the health and appearance of the mouth as well as making eating easier, and in time contributing to an improvement in their general condition.

As well as the local features associated with oral conditions the nurse must not forget that some of the diseases will give rise to a systemic illness characterized by fever, headache and malaise. Symptoms should be treated as they arise, as well as the underlying pathological cause.

CHAPTER 3

The Oesophagus

The oesophagus is a development of the distal part of the foregut between the pharynx and diaphragm. In the embryo elongation takes place rapidly and there is a temporary obliteration of the lumen. Later, recanalization takes place and the columnar cells which originally lined the lumen are replaced by a stratified squamous epithelium. Failure of the oesophagus to recanalize is the cause of some of the congenital anomalies which will be described later. A groove appears in the floor of the foregut and this later converts into a tube and becomes the larynx and trachea, a bud grows out from either side and these eventually form the lungs; the position of these structures results in a very close anatomical relationship with the oesophagus.

In the adult then, the oesophagus extends from the lower border of the cricoid cartilage to the cardiac orifice of the stomach, a distance of 25 cm. It is a muscular tube, the upper two-thirds being striated muscle tissue and the lower third unstriated and therefore resembling the remainder of the gut musculature. The squamous epithelial lining is continuous with that of the mouth, and below this is a submucous layer containing glands. The whole is surrounded by a connective tissue sheath. The oesophagus commences in the median plane, then deviates slightly to the left as it approaches the thoracic inlet, returning to the midline at the level of the fifth thoracic vertebra, from whence it passes downwards, forwards and then to the left to pass through the oesophageal opening in the diaphragm where it comes to rest in a groove on the posterior surface of the left lobe of the liver. In this area it is covered anteriorly and on its left aspect by peritoneum. As the oesophagus passes through the thorax it is crossed anteriorly by the trachea and left bronchus, and is separated from the left atrium of the heart by the pericardium. In the neck the oesophagus is flanked on either side by the common carotid arteries and recurrent laryngeal nerves, whilst the trachea and thyroid gland lie anteriorly and the lower cervical vertebrae and prevertebral fascia are on its posterior aspect.

The oesophagus obtains its blood supply from the inferior thyroid arteries, branches from the descending aorta and the left gastric artery. Venous drainage of the upper part is into the inferior thyroid veins and of the lower part into the left gastric vein and from the thoracic portion into the azygos vein. An anastomosis forms between the azygos vein which is part of the systemic circulation and the venous tributaries of the left gastric vein, this latter belonging to the portal circulation. This factor is of great importance especially in conditions such as portal hypertension where these veins become distended and varicose, leading to rupture and consequently a large haemorrhage. The two branches of the vagus nerve form a plexus on the surface of the lower portion of the oesophagus, the right vagus nerve lying posteriorly and the left anteriorly. Surrounding the oesophagus is a lymphatic plexus which conveys lymph into the posterior mediastinal nodes, from which it is drained into both the nodes surrounding the left gastric vessels and the supraclavicular nodes.

Dysphagia

Pain and difficulty in swallowing may result from any lesion in the mouth or pharynx because these interfere with the mobility of the tongue which is actively concerned in the process of swallowing (page 33). Similarly, conditions either in or adjacent to the oesophagus may also give rise to the same symptom, and some medical conditions such as iron deficiency anaemia. Often the patient complains that food sticks at a particular point, and this may help to localize the area of the lesion, often due to carcinoma. Trauma to the oesophagus such as may result from swallowing a corrosive substance will usually cause structure and dysphagia. Dysphagia may also present as a complication of peptic ulceration where this occurs in the oesophagus, or be due to a foreign body which has become arrested in its passage through to the stomach. Hiatus hernia and achalasia of the cardia are also causes of dysphagia.

Conditions which arise adjacent to the oesophagus may also cause dysphagia due to the pressure that they exert on this structure. These include enlarged mediastinal lymph nodes, aortic aneurysm, hypertrophy of the left atrium resulting from mitral stenosis and pericarditis. Diagnosis of the cause of dysphagia may be assisted by a barium swallow, followed by a barium meal if no cause is found above the level of the diaphragm.

CONGENITAL ANOMALIES

Atresia

The most common abnormality is atresia often accompanied by a tracheo-oesophageal fistula; in the majority of cases it is the lower portion of the oesophagus which communicates with the trachea. Oesophageal atresia occurs in one of its forms in about one in three thousand births, either as complete absence of the oesophagus, or a simple atresia or complicated by fistula formation. It is a very serious situation and one which must be diagnosed within twenty-four hours of birth so that life-saving surgery may be attempted. Several factors are often associated with this condition, and the skilled midwife will bear these in mind at the time of the baby's birth and first examination, namely the presence of hydramnios in the antenatal period, followed by the birth of a premature baby which has frequent cyanotic attacks in the first few hours due to an excessive production of mucus from the respiratory tract. If the baby is given a feed it is likely to cough, choke and become cyanosed. Diagnosis is made by passing a fine rigid oesophageal tube through the nostril into the stomach; if atresia is present the passage of the tube will be arrested about 10 cm from the nose. Confirmation is then made by taking a plain X-ray film of the chest and abdomen which will indicate areas of collapsed lung tissue. The presence of gas in the stomach and intestines is indicative of a fistula.

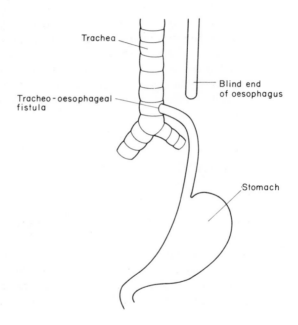

Trachea

Tracheo-oesophageal
fistula

Blind end
of oesophagus

Stomach

Fig. 11. *Oesophageal atresia with tracheo-oesophageal fistula.*

Treatment

Surgery should be undertaken immediately to reconstruct the oesophagus and close the fistula; this is achieved through a right thoracotomy incision. Occasionally it is not possible to repair the oesophagus adequately at this stage and a gastrostomy may need to be made through which the baby can be fed until it becomes bigger and stronger. At a suitable time a more extensive operation is carried out using part of the colon to replace the deficient oesophagus. A fine oesophageal tube (size 4 EG/10 FG) is left in place so that feeds can be given; occasionally a gastrostomy is undertaken as an emergency measure. Whilst awaiting operation the baby must not be given anything by mouth and must be constantly observed so that mucus may be aspirated when produced. An incubator should be available for the nursing of this baby. The paediatrician will have made a thorough examination of the baby to elicit other abnormalities such as congenital heart disease and imperforate anus which may occur in association. The parents of the baby will naturally be most concerned, and their consent for operation must be obtained and facilities given for emergency baptism if they should so wish. Prophylactic antibiotics will usually be commenced because of the risk of respiratory infection, and a specimen of blood should be obtained for cross-matching as transfusion may be necessary. The doctor may set up an intravenous infusion using a scalp vein if possible, so that fluids may be given and any electrolyte imbalance corrected.

Post-operative nursing care

The baby will be nursed in an incubator, where the minimum of clothes may be worn, whilst the temperature and humidity are carefully controlled. Oxygen may be administered by running this into the incubator, but should only be given if the baby cannot maintain a satisfactory colour without it. Aspiration of mucus using gentle suction should be carried out as required, and observations made on the baby's colour and temperature, together with the passing of meconium and urine. The nurse will need to devise some form of restraint so that the baby does not interfere with the intravenous cannula, as the infusion will probably remain in progress for twenty-four hours. Feeding will be by the oesophageal tube, a small quantity of water being given as the first feed in order to test the adequacy of the anastomosis. If all is well, subsequent feeds may be of milk, gradually increasing the amount given until a normal feeding regimen is achieved. After a few days the tube will be removed and oral feeding commenced. Sutures in the thoracotomy wound will be removed on about the eighth post-operative day, and probably no further dressings will be necessary. By this time the baby (unless it is very premature) will no longer need to be nursed in the incubator, and provided his colour and temperature control are satisfactory he may be dressed and nursed in the usual way.

Stenosis

Congenital stenosis of the oesophagus is far less common than atresia, and usually does not give rise to symptoms until a mixed diet is introduced when the baby is a few months old. Withholding solid foods for a little longer may enable the condition to be spontaneously corrected, otherwise the use of dilators will be necessary.

FOREIGN BODIES IN THE OESOPHAGUS

This accident may occur in young children who are likely to swallow toys or buttons which become lodged in the oesophagus. It can also occur in the adult and may be due to a broken denture, safety pin or similar object. Removal of the foreign body must be undertaken as soon as possible, the object being extracted with special forceps passed through an oesophagoscope whilst the patient is anaesthetized. Previously an X-ray will reveal any object which is radio-opaque, or a small barium meal may need to be given.

ACHALASIA OF THE CARDIA

This term is used to describe an acquired condition in which the bolus of food fails to be propelled through the lower part of the oesophagus. Many theories have been put forward as to the cause of this, but there is evidence to suppose that some neuromuscular imbalance is present which causes abnormal muscular action; this results in large quantities of food being dammed up in the oesophagus which eventually undergoes dilatation. The patient complains that food sticks and this may be accompanied by pain. At first the symptoms are infrequent, but after months or years they become more severe with a marked increase in the amount of pain due to oesophagitis. The patient may have found that a change to a more fluid diet, or the drinking of large quantities of fluid during the course of a meal may have given some relief in the early stages.

A barium swallow will reveal the dilated oesophagus which tapers at the lower end. Prior to this the patient should have had a fluid diet for two days and then an oesophageal washout immediately prior to the investigation. An oesophagoscopy should also be done, so that biopsy may be carried out in order to exclude carcinoma. Treatment of this condition must be either conservative or operative; drugs have proved to be of no value.

Conservative treatment

A rubber bougie which has been weighted with mercury is passed daily by the patient into the oesophagus. This should produce sufficient dilatation to allow food to be taken during the next twenty-four hours. This technique produces favourable results but many patients would prefer operative treatment.

Surgical treatment

The lower end of the oesophagus and the cardiac sphincter may be stretched by the surgeon's finger introduced through an opening in the stomach, or Heller's operation may be performed. This operation is now the treatment of choice as the results are good. It is based on the operation of pyloromyotomy performed for congenital hypertrophic pyloric stenosis (page 69) in which the muscle layer is divided down to the submucus layer; this relieves the constriction.

TRAUMA AND INFLAMMATION OF THE OESOPHAGUS

Ulceration of the oesophagus usually follows the swallowing of corrosive fluids. At first gross oedema obstructs the oesophagus and this is later replaced by fibrous tissue forming a stricture. As the passage of a tube would probably perforate the oesophagus, a gastrostomy will need to be performed in the initial stages so that feeding can be maintained. Treatment of the resulting stricture may be achieved by the frequent passing of bougies, or later the patient may need to undergo an operation where a portion of colon is used to replace the damaged length of oesophagus. Immediate repair of the oesophagus will be necessary if it has been severed during wounding with a knife. Oesophagitis will occur as a result of damage by corrosive poisons or from gastric reflux in conditions such as hiatus hernia. It may also result from radiotherapy to the area, and very occasionally as a complication of miliary tuberculosis and syphilis. Infection occurring in the oesophagus is likely to be due to an extension of a monilial infection from the mouth, and will be treated accordingly.

OESOPHAGEAL VARICES

Oesophageal varices are likely to occur in portal hypertension, in which relief of the hypertension is partly achieved by the setting up of a collateral circulation to drain venous blood from the liver and convey it to the azygos vein draining the oesophagus. This blood flow is possible owing to the anastomosis of the portal and systemic circulations at this point. The oesophageal veins become dilated and varicose and are likely to rupture giving rise to a sudden, dangerous haemorrhage superimposed on existing severe liver disease. Immediate steps must be taken to control the bleeding and transfuse the patient. A Sengstaken tube may be passed into the stomach and inflated so that pressure is exerted on the bleeding vessels. Such a tube consists of three lumens bound together. One tube forms a means of aspirating the stomach and also a means by which feeds may be given, a second tube ends in a small wide balloon which when it is inflated (after the tube has passed into the stomach) can be pulled back against the cardia of the stomach to hold the tube in place and prevents its removal, whilst the third lumen connects to a long balloon which fits the oesophagus when inflated and thus exerts pressure at its lower end. The tube remains in place for forty-eight hours or even longer if bleeding is not controlled, in which case it should be deflated for a time and then reinflated. Surgery in the form of a portacaval anastomosis may need to be carried out for repeated haemorrhage from oesophageal varices, but the decision to operate depends amongst other things on the extent of hepatic damage (*see* Chapter 5).

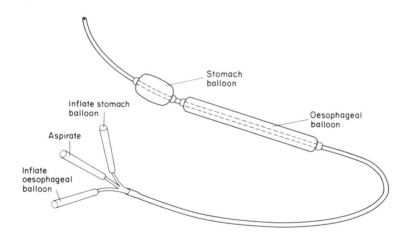

Fig. 12. *Sengstaken tube.*

Hiatus hernia

See Chapter 11.

NEOPLASTIC CONDITIONS

Carcinoma is the most common of malignant tumours of the oesophagus; benign tumours are rarely seen. Two histological types of tumour may occur, the squamous cell carcinoma occurring in the upper part of the oesophagus, and the adenocarcinoma at the lower end where the epithelium changes to the columnar type found in the stomach. Either type may spread by direct invasion or through the blood and lymphatic vessels, eventually giving rise to fistulae between the oesophagus and trachea, bronchi or aorta, or else invade the stomach and liver.

Carcinoma of the oesophagus is rare in younger persons. More often it occurs in men in their sixties and seventies, and is thought to be associated with a heavy consumption of alcohol, smoking, and malignant conditions occurring in other parts of the gastrointestinal tract. Symptoms are usually few at first, the chief being dysphagia, which may progress to a stage where only liquids can be swallowed. In the later stages of the condition retrosternal pain is experienced, and cough may be present especially if the carcinoma has become invasive and fistula formation has occurred. Continual loss of weight is a feature of the condition. Diagnosis is confirmed by barium swallow, which shows an irregular constriction of the oesophagus, oesophagoscopy, biopsy and cytology.

Treatment

Treatment may be by either surgery or radiotherapy, the choice depending on the location of the tumour and how far advanced it is. Growths in the upper and lower thirds are best treated by operation, whereas the middle third because of its close proximity to the heart may be treated by radiotherapy; this is achieved by the use of the linear accelerator. In the event of severe oesophagitis surgery may be required to insert a gastrostomy tube so that feeding may be maintained whilst the radiotherapy treatment continues.

Surgery may take the form of an excision of the affected part of the oesophagus or a by-pass operation. For either of these operations a length of colon (ascending and transverse) or jejunum is brought up from the abdomen complete with its blood supply and this is anastomosed to the upper oesophagus and the stomach. When surgery of this nature is not possible a PVC or nylon tube may be implanted into the oesophagus to dilate it sufficiently to allow the passage of food; this proves satisfactory for several months but in time will cause oesophagitis, necrosis and infection. Whatever form of treatment is decided upon the patient requires a high protein and high calorie diet in order to replace some of the weight that has been lost. Anaemia also needs to be corrected.

Nursing care

Carcinoma or trauma of the oesophagus necessitate very skilled nursing care being given to the patient, principally because of the close proximity of the oesophagus to the trachea and diaphragm which makes respiratory complications a very real hazard. When carcinoma is present it must also be remembered that the patient is usually elderly and by no means in a fit condition to undergo extensive surgery. Operations of this nature are likely to result in considerable blood loss and so transfusion is necessary. Operations to repair, reconstruct or by-pass the oesophagus may be carried out through a thoracic or abdominal incision or there may be a combined approach. Where the chest has been opened the surgeon may close it completely (this is usually the case in babies) or may leave a catheter in place attached to an underwater seal drainage apparatus in order to allow the escape of both fluid and air from the pleural space, and enable the lung to reinflate. In either case there is the risk of atelectasis, mainly of the basal lobe of the lung, or the complications of haemothorax and pleural effusion.

Underwater seal drainage is a procedure in which the catheter with its tip in the pleural space is held in place by a skin suture, and then attached by a length of extension tubing to an angled glass tube passing through a tightly fitting bung into a sterile drainage jar. Also passing through the bung is another short angled tube which is open to the atmosphere. The drainage tube must be long enough to reach almost to the bottom of the jar to allow about 2·5 cm of the measured sterile fluid placed in the jar to pass up the tube. As the patient breathes in the level of the fluid at the base of the drainage tube moves up the tube a short distance, returning to its original position on expiration; this feature is often termed 'swinging'. Fluid in the pleural space may drain out through this tube and air can be expelled when the patient coughs. Both of these measures help to restore the normal negative pressure in the pleural space and allow the lung to re-expand; this may take only a few hours or several days to achieve. Sometimes two intrapleural drainage tubes are used, each attached to its own drainage jar, the basal tube draining fluid and the apical tube, air. Removal of the tube is carried out when the doctor is sure that lung expansion has taken place, an indication being the cessation of drainage, very little 'swing' in the tube, good respiratory movements on the part of the patient and a satisfactory chest X-ray film report. Whilst caring for the underwater seal drainage the nurse must remember that the drainage jar (which normally hangs below the bed) must not be lifted to bed level or above else the fluid will syphon back along the tubing into the pleural space. Also that the apparatus must never be disconnected unless the chest catheter is securely clamped, and that frequent observations must be made to see that the drainage is continuing satisfactorily and no kinking of the tubing has occurred. The amount of drainage can be estimated (usually twice a day) when the drainage jar is replaced, the nurse maintaining strict asepsis throughout this procedure.

As a complication of the abdominal approach the patient is at risk of developing a paralytic ileus, and possibly peritonitis. Whatever route is used complications may arise at the site of the anastomosis. Leakage here may cause infection in the mediastinum which can progress to the formation of a mediastinal abscess. Bearing these complications in mind the nurse must encourage her patient to do frequent deep breathing movements of the chest and to cough up secretions; in this aspect she will be assisted by the physiotherapist. If an operation has been performed to remove and replace part of the oesophagus with a length of colon, then it is likely that part of the larynx and trachea will also have been removed which will mean that a tracheostomy will have been performed and in the immediate post-operative period regular tracheal suction will be

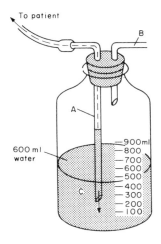

Fig. 13. *Underwater seal drainage apparatus; (a) tube connected to drainage tubing; (b) air inlet tube; (c) water seal.*

necessary. As infection is such a danger to operations on the oesophagus careful attention to oral hygiene is essential both before and after surgery. Antibiotic mouthwashes may be given to be swallowed, this being the only fluid at first to pass directly in contact with the anastomosis, the patient being discouraged from swallowing saliva or other mouthwash. Also to prevent infection, the area round the anastomosis is usually drained for several days to prevent the accumulation of a fluid medium suitable for bacterial growth.

As has already been suggested the patient will need a high protein and high calorie diet in order to regain weight; in some operations on the oesophagus a nasogastric catheter will be introduced so that all feeds can be given by this route to allow the anastomosis to heal without food continually passing over it. For some patients it may be necessary to perform a gastrostomy and the nurse will need to give the feeds through this tube and probably in time can encourage the patient to do them for himself. The patient may be permitted to chew a pleasant flavoured substance such as chewing gum (provided he can be relied on not to swallow it) as this will encourage the flow of digestive juices at the start of the feed and also help to keep the mouth clean. For details concerning the care of the gastrostomy tube and the method of feeding see page 13.

CHAPTER 4

The Stomach

Development of the stomach

The characteristic J-shaped stomach forms early in fetal life from
the latter part of the foregut before it merges with the midgut at the
point of entry of the bile ducts into the duodenum. The gut wall
grows rapidly and this results in obliteration of the lumen, which

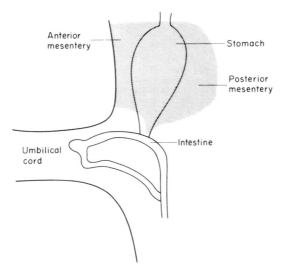

Fig. 14. *Early development of lesser and greater omentum.*

59

later undergoes a process of recanalization. During development the stomach rotates, but before it does so a simple tissue forming a midline partition extends from the lesser curvature of the stomach to the anterior body wall. As the liver and bile ducts develop they grow into this partition dividing it into regions; the part between the lesser curvature of the stomach and the dorsal aspect of the liver will eventually become that part of the peritoneum known as the lesser omentum. The free border of this structure supports the hepatic artery, portal vein and bile duct where they enter and leave the liver at the porta hepatis. The lesser omentum is a double sheet of peritoneum which encloses the stomach and reforms at the greater curvature to continue as the greater omentum. Growth of the

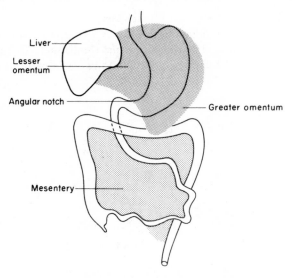

Fig. 15. *Rotation of stomach completed.*

stomach and its adjacent organs causes the former to rotate, and as it does so an alteration in the plane of the lesser omentum occurs resulting in the formation of the lesser sac—an extensive pouch lying behind the stomach and lesser omentum, bounded by the spleen to the left and communicating with the main peritoneal cavity through the foramen of Winslow to the right. Rotation of the gut and formation of the lesser sac results in the greater curvature of the stomach now coming to lie towards the left (having previously been posterior) and the duodenum is swung round to the right. The vagus nerves rotate with the stomach, hence the left vagus nerve tends to supply the area of the stomach over the lesser curvature. The mesentery of the duodenum now fuses with the dorsal parietal peritoneum and this organ becomes retro-peritoneal. The fact that the lesser sac is in communication with the main peritoneal cavity at the foramen of Winslow will make it possible for a loop of gut to pass through the foramen and become strangulated by the edges of the opening. Decompression of the gut is necessary in order to

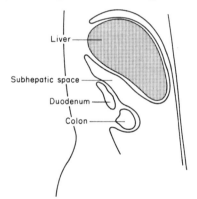

Fig. 16. *Subhepatic space.*

secure its release. The peritoneal attachments of the liver cause the formation of several potential spaces. In relation to the stomach the most important are the right and left subhepatic spaces, which are in communication with each other through the foramen of Winslow and allow fluid to enter the latter from a perforated stomach. The right subhepatic space communicates with the right subphrenic space and in this area abscess formation may result from a perforated peptic ulcer.

Gastric function

An eminent surgeon once described the stomach as 'a gland with a cavity'. This gland in fact consists of some thirty-five million branched secreting glands, about every four of which empty their contents into one gastric pit. On inspection the gastric mucosa is studded with the openings of these pits, the mucous membrane being covered by a slimy mucus which is secreted by cells in the glands, together with those lining the gastric pits and the cells of the surface epithelium. The glands in the cardia and body of the stomach possess oxyntic cells which produce hydrochloric acid, peptic cells producing pepsinogen, and other cells nearer the neck of the glands which probably produce the intrinsic factor. Around the entrance of the oesophagus into the stomach and in the pyloric antrum are to be found glands which secrete mucus only, giving rise to a slightly alkaline medium which buffers the hydrochloric acid as it passes through to the duodenum. These glands are longer than those elsewhere in the stomach and tend to be coiled, and the mucus secreting cells are constantly undergoing replacement, being renewed about every two days. This viscid fluid bathes the mucosal surface of the stomach and performs an important protective role against chemical and mechanical injury.

Gastric juice

On average two to three litres of gastric juice are secreted each twenty-four hours, and whilst the stomach is actively secreting, the mucosa becomes red and swollen and the mucus thicker and difficult to remove. The high concentration of hydrochloric acid gives the juice an average range of pH $1 \cdot 6-2$. This will of course vary due to a number of factors including the age of the individual (for a few hours after birth the pH is about 5, but quickly falls to around pH 2) the presence of food in the stomach, and conditions which affect the release of hydrochloric acid when the level may be as high as pH 8 in cases of achlorhydria. The hydrochloric acid causes pepsinogen to be converted to pepsin which breaks protein to proteoses or peptones, the subsequent breakdown to amino acids occurring in the small intestine by the action of pancreatic and intestinal enzymes. It is not strictly necessary for protein digestion to be started in the stomach, as has been shown following removal of the stomach for malignancy, when total protein digestion has taken place adequately in the duodenum. Pepsinogen is excreted in the urine, the level showing a marked rise in conditions of duodenal ulceration. In babies the action of pepsin on the clotting of milk is augmented by the enzyme rennin, but even if this is present in adult gastric secretion it is inactive due to the low pH prevailing. Lipase, present in gastric juice is a fat-splitting enzyme. The intrinsic factor is concerned with the uptake of vitamin B_{12}, and following an injection of histamine the output is more than doubled, a factor which is made use of in the augmented histamine test (*see* page 66). Antihistamine drugs when applied to the gastric mucosa cause inhibition of acid secretion, but have no effect on the pepsinogen producing cells.

Control of gastric secretion

Secretion of gastric juice is partly under the control of the nervous system as a result of vagus nerve activity. This is an important factor in the amount of acid and pepsinogen produced, as well as encouraging the release of gastrin in the pyloric antrum and conditioning the oxyntic cells to its effects. Distension of the pyloric antrum in association with vagal stimulation and a rise in the pH of the gastric contents is responsible for the release of gastrin. This histamine-containing hormone stimulates further production of hydrochloric acid and pepsinogen as well as increasing gastrointestinal motility. It will be noted that the nervous and hormonal aspects of control of gastric secretion are very closely linked. Gastric secretion is inhibited partly by the fall in the pH of the gastric contents reaching the pyloric antrum, and also when they pass through into the duodenum thus lowering the pH there. The presence of fat in a meal reduces the motility of the entire stomach and also affects secretion; this will delay emptying of the stomach.

The hormone enterogastrone, produced in the duodenum when food enters which contains a high fat content, is thought to have an inhibitory effect on gastric secretion and motility. Other endocrines exert an influence on the function of the gastric mucosa, chief of which are the hormones released by the anterior lobe of the pituitary gland. Evidence of this is seen in conditions such as Addison's disease where the secretion of adrenal cortical hormones is reduced and the gastric musoca atrophies; or in the reverse situation, following prolonged administration of corticosteroids which cause a marked increase in gastric secretion giving rise to one of the complications of this type of therapy.

Gastric movements

As food enters and fills the stomach the smooth muscle fibres increase in length and allow the walls to relax, particularly along the greater curvature and in the fundus, and the organ distends. Contractions of the circular muscle fibres cause peristaltic waves which start in the body of the stomach and travel towards the pylorus. The most active part of the stomach is the lower third, the other two-thirds acting as a storage organ where food is softened and mixed with the gastric juice. Churning of the food occurs in the pyloric antrum, and from time to time food is passed on into the duodenum. Drugs such as atropine and adrenaline block the vagus nerve and have the effect of reducing gastric motility, as does the operation of vagotomy which results in delay in emptying of the stomach contents. The narrow lumen of the pyloric antrum helps prevent the reflux of duodenal content into the stomach (although this does occur) and also causes large particles of food to be retained in the stomach until they have been adequately churned and mixed with the gastric juice. Gastric peristalsis is reduced by the presence in the duodenum of carbohydrates and fats, probably brought about by the action of the hormone enterogastrone released from the wall of the duodenum. Food normally starts to leave the stomach within ten minutes of its ingestion, the gastric emptying time (that is the time interval between the ingestion of a meal and when the last portion has left the stomach) varies with the constituents of the meal and the emotional state of the individual. Starchy foods leave the stomach quickly, leafy vegetables are slow, and fatty foods have the longest delay. The nurse should remember that in a state of fear all gastric functions are delayed and a meal may remain undigested in the stomach for twelve hours or more. Conversely, in excitement the rate at which the stomach empties is increased.

Vomiting

The act of vomiting is brought about by the action of the respiratory and abdominal muscles, not by peristaltic waves occurring in the stomach. The stomach contracts at the angular notch and this has the effect of forcing the pyloric contents back into the relaxed body and fundus. The glottis closes following a deep inspiration and the soft palate rises to occlude the nasopharynx and prevent vomit entering the nose. Violent contraction of the abdominal muscles causes a sharp increase in intra-abdominal pressure and this forces the gastric contents through the cardiac orifice and along the oesophagus into the mouth. In the unconscious person the glottis may not close completely and there is a risk of vomit being inhaled into the lungs. Prior to the act of vomiting retching may have occurred; this is a state where the stomach is repeatedly compressed by violent contractions of the abdominal muscles and diaphragm, and is usually accompanied by nausea. Pallor, sweating, salivation and a slowing of the heart rate may also occur. It has been shown that there is a sensory area in the medulla of the brain which initiates vomiting following stimulation, mainly by the vagus nerve endings. This centre also receives impulses from the higher centres, and this accounts for vomiting occurring following visual stimulation, for example the sight of one person being seasick may cause another to do likewise. Distension of the gut and gall bladder, or irritation of the intestinal mucosa and occlusion of the coronary blood vessels cause stimuli to pass to the centre of the medulla and account for the initiation of vomiting in these conditions. Other stimuli which may result in vomiting include severe pain, raised intracranial pressure and feelings of disgust.

Vomiting can be induced as a first aid measure when it is necessary to empty the stomach quickly, by irritating the back of the throat with the finger. The use of salt water or similar fluid as an emetic is to be discouraged. Conversely, the medullary centre can be made insensitive to stimuli by the giving of anti-emetic drugs such as nitrazepam, and thus vomiting can be prevented.

Gastric investigations

In order to obtain a diagnosis the doctor may request a number of investigations to be carried out. The nurse must ensure that the patient has been given an adequate explanation of what the test involves so that his cooperation is obtained at the outset, and that the correct preparation is given to enable a successful outcome at the first attempt. The principles underlying the various tests are included here; for more detail regarding the preparation of the patient and subsequent care the reader should refer to Chapter 14.

Gastric secretion
Gastric juice may be obtained for investigation by passing a Ryle's tube into the stomach and aspirating the total juice (resting juice) present after a period of starvation. Examination may then be carried out in respect of the acid level and enzyme content. Abnormalities may be present in the juice such as excessive mucus or blood, found sometimes in conditions of gastric ulcer or carcinoma of the stomach.

Augmented histamine test
A test meal may also be undertaken to investigate the quality of the gastric juice and the response of the stomach to the intake of food. The procedure for this test is to first empty the stomach by aspirating the gastric juice through a Ryle's tube, and then to give a 'meal'

in the form of an injection of histamine or insulin. In normal circumstances this would provoke an increase in the amount of acid produced. As histamine may cause unpleasant side effects it is customary to give an antihistamine drug by intramuscular injection thirty minutes prior to injecting the histamine. Samples of gastric juice are aspirated at intervals (usually over a period of one hour). The results of investigations on the juice should give the doctor an indication of the amount of secretion produced over a given period of time, the normal rise and decline in the amount of acid released following the 'meal', and the length of time the stomach takes to empty. The term 'meal' has been retained for this investigation although the factor used is injected into the patient; prior to this type of test the patient was asked to drink 50 ml of 7% alcohol or a measured quantity of gruel as the 'meal'.

Histalog test

Betazole hydrochloride (Histalog) is an oral preparation used in a dose of 50 mg. The results obtained correspond closely to those following an augmented histamine test, which however has the advantage that it does not give rise to unpleasant side effects.

Pentagastrin test

This is a synthetic preparation of gastrin and can be given by either slow intravenous infusion or a single subcutaneous injection. It produces maximum stimulation after ten minutes and gives rise to few side effects.

Diagnex test

In this test a dye (Azure A) is given to the patient one hour after stimulation of gastric secretion by betazole hydrochloride (Histalog) or caffeine benzoate. After two hours the urine is collected and if acid is being secreted by the stomach this will have caused absorption of the dye to take place which will subsequently be excreted in the urine, colouring it blue.

Barium meal

A contrast X-ray in the form of a barium meal is frequently used to assist in a diagnosis of gastric or duodenal ulcer. The patient drinks a quantity of barium sulphate and the movements of the stomach are watched on the screen by the radiologist, who then indicates the most appropriate times for the radiographer to take the X-ray films. If an ulcer is present it may well show as a crater filled with barium extending down into the stomach wall. This investigation is particularly useful in the diagnosis of ulcers situated on the lesser curvature of the stomach.

Gastroscopy and biopsy

Direct viewing of the gastric mucosa is possible with the aid of a gastroscope introduced into the stomach through the mouth and oesophagus. The partially flexible metal tube carrying a light at its tip has largely been replaced by the gastro-fibrescope, a highly sophisticated instrument made of hundreds of glass fibres which allow for considerable mobility at the tip, and either side or end viewing. This delicate instrument enables the operator to alter the position of the gastroscope in order to view all regions of the stomach, to obtain a specimen of the mucosa (biopsy), to introduce fluid into the stomach and aspirate the gastric juice, as well as to attach a small camera to take still or ciné colour photographs, the latter being undertaken by an assistant who views the stomach through an additional channel of the fibrescope. Benign and malignant ulceration of the stomach wall can be differentiated by this method, the former appearing as a greyish white slough on the mucosa, whilst the latter has a less regular appearance with nodules in the surrounding tissue.

Cytology

Examination of cells from the stomach wall may enable the cytologist to make an early diagnosis in conditions such as carcinoma of the stomach and thus make treatment more successful. Cells are obtained either from 'gastric washings', that is aspirating the gastric juice through a Ryle's tube having introduced a measured amount of fluid into the stomach, or by 'brushings', where an attachment to the gastro-fibrescope allows cells to be swept off the mucosa and collected for investigation. New methods of gastric investigation are constantly being sought, and the time is not too far distant when the patient will only be required to swallow a small capsule which is capable of transmitting ultrasonic waves to be viewed on a small screen situated in a laboratory some distance away. This will give amongst other information the pressure in the lumen of the gut, and the pH content at various levels of the gastrointestinal tract as the capsule passes through. This will undoubtedly make some aspects of gastric investigation a simpler and more pleasant procedure for the patient.

CONGENITAL ANOMALIES

Congenital hypertrophic pyloric stenosis

This is one of the commonest congenital malformations of the gastrointestinal tract, occurring approximately 1 in 350 live births. Most commonly it is the firstborn and a male child which has this condition. There is some evidence to suggest that genetic factors have a bearing on the incidence. The circular muscle fibres in the pyloric region are grossly hypertrophied (rarely the longitudinal fibres are affected) which narrows the pyloric lumen although the mucosa remains unchanged. Characteristically the signs are not evident until the baby is about three weeks old, but onset may be at any time before the baby is three months old when spontaneous remission of symptoms occurs. In the early stages vomiting may occur once or twice a day, but as time progresses this happens on each occasion the baby is fed. Vomiting occurs with considerable force, being described as projectile, distinguishing it from the normal possetingthat many babies do at the end of a feed. At first the baby will appear hungry and demand the feed to be repeated, but as dehydration progresses rapid weight loss occurs, the urine output becomes scanty and the baby is apathetic, listless and gravely ill.

Diagnosis is made partly on the history obtained from the

mother, together with the paediatrician palpating a hard 'tumour' which is the pyloric muscles in spasm, felt whilst the baby is in the process of taking a feed. Waves of peristalsis passing across the abdomen may also be noted. The majority of infants require surgery to correct the condition, although mild cases may sometimes be helped by giving an anticholinergic drug in the form of atropine methonitrate (Eumydrin) 1–3 drops of a 0·6% solution before each feed. It is important that no changes are made in the type of feed the baby is having, and when hospital admission is necessary arrangements will need to be made to enable the mother who is breast feeding to accompany her baby. Once surgery has been decided upon, the doctor may delay operation for a few hours until the general condition of the baby has been improved by the giving of intravenous fluids enabling the electrolyte balance to be corrected. Pre-operative treatment usually takes the form of a stomach washout using tap or sterile water to remove any mucus or milk curds. The baby is then placed on a cruciform splint, care being taken to see that the limbs are adequately protected and kept warm, leaving just the abdomen exposed. Some surgeons prefer to do the operation under local anaesthesia in which case the baby may be given chloral hydrate before going to the theatre. The operation of pyloromyotomy (Ramstedt's operation) consists of removing a wedge of circular muscle tissue at the pylorus, down as far as the submucous layer but not involving it; this simply allows for distension of the narrowed lumen of the pylorus into the space previously occupied by the muscle. As this is a relatively avascular area of the stomach no suturing is required. The abdominal wall is closed in

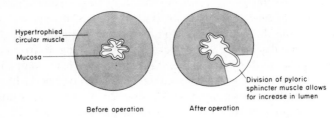

Hypertrophied circular muscle

Mucosa

Division of pyloric sphincter muscle allows for increase in lumen

Before operation   After operation

Fig. 17. *Before and after pyloromyotomy.*

layers and usually a continuous nylon suture closes the skin. If a local anaesthetic is given, a nurse needs to sit near the head of the baby, so that when the surgeon starts the closure of the peritoneum (and not before) she may offer a dummy to quieten the baby if he is restless at this stage. The baby's temperature must be monitored continuously during the operation as hypothermia quickly develops at this age. Feeding is usually commenced within two to four hours of completion of the operation, starting with a small quantity (about 10 ml) of glucose in water, and then introducing diluted milk feeds six hours post-operatively. The strength and amount of the feed can then be increased each time provided there is no further vomiting until a normal feeding regimen is re-established after about twenty-four hours. If the baby is breast fed, then it may be put to the breast four hours after operation, the mother being advised to feed for about two minutes at each breast to start with, and gradually to increase the time at each successive feed. Provided the baby is taking feeds without vomiting and appears well, he will probably be discharged from hospital on about the third or fourth post-operative day, to return on the eighth day for removal of the suture. Complications following this operation are uncommon, the majority of babies quickly regain the lost weight and appear to thrive.

TRAUMA

Foreign bodies

A variety of objects may reach the stomach, in some instances these are deliberatedly swallowed. They include safety pins (open or closed), buttons and small toys, and the majority will show on an X-ray film of the abdomen. Provided the object is small and has no sharp features it may be allowed to continue its passage through the gastrointestinal tract, observation being made that it has completed the journey. Sharp objects may cause trauma to the stomach; therefore gastrotomy should be performed to remove the object and repair the stomach wall. If trauma has not occurred then the surgeon may decide to wait and observe the progress of the object through the remainder of the gut having taken the precaution of giving cotton wool sandwiches to the patient. If the object fails to move on then operation for its removal will be necessary.

INFLAMMATORY AND INFECTIVE CONDITIONS

Gastritis

This is a rather vague term used to describe a number of conditions where definite changes in the gastric mucosa have occurred, often as a result of ingestion of harmful substances or organisms. Acute gastritis may be subdivided as follows.

Simple exogenous

This is a condition resulting from exposure to a harmful agent such as alcohol, staphylococcal food poisoning or salicylates; in the latter instance it is estimated that about 70% of persons taking this form of therapy for conditions such as rheumatoid arthritis lose up to 10 ml per day as occult bleeding from a damaged mucosa. Features of this condition are epigastric discomfort which may progress to actual pain, nausea and possible vomiting occurring soon after a meal. The patient may be pale, sweating and possibly pyrexial with a raised pulse rate. On examination the gastric mucosa appears hyperaemic and erosions are present with a purulent exudate. The condition usually improves rapidly and the mucosa reverts to its normal features in a short time.

Acute systemic infections

These infections may give rise to acute gastritis, where the toxic agent produced during a febrile illness is responsible for causing necrosis at the neck of the gastric glands and erosions similar to those just described. Treatment is by giving small meals, bland in composition, plenty of fluids and attention to the underlying illness. These measures will effect an improvement in the condition.

Acute corrosive gastritis

This condition occurs as a result of ingesting a strong acid or alkali such as sulphuric or nitric acid or sodium hydroxide. In this instance there is widespread necrosis and softening of the mucosa which may lead to sloughing of large areas of the stomach wall. The patient immediately complains of severe pain in the mouth and throat, accompanied by burning substernal pain. Vomiting may occur. There is rapid onset of shock and collapse. Treatment of this condition is to convey the patient to hospital urgently. In the meantime it is unwise to give an emetic or attempt to pass a tube to empty the stomach; water or milk may be given by mouth to help dilute the poison provided the casualty is conscious. Pain may be relieved by injection of an analgesic, and respiratory or cardiac resuscitation may be necessary. Once in hospital the patient will probably require a tracheostomy and extensive plastic repair of the damaged tissues, whilst nutrition is maintained through a nasogastric or gastrostomy tube after an initial period of intravenous feeding. It cannot be stressed too frequently the need for great care to be exercised over the storage and availability of such corrosive poisons, in order that an accident such as this is prevented, particularly where young children are concerned.

Acute suppurative gastritis

This condition results from the direct invasion of the stomach wall by pyogenic bacteria, usually the haemolytic streptococcus, into an already ulcerated area such as results from carcinoma, the whole giving rise to the formation of abscesses. The onset is sudden with severe epigastric pain, nausea, vomiting, pyrexia and collapse, the condition being compared with the features of an acute abdomen. Partial or total gastrectomy will be necessary together with the use of antibiotics; even so the mortality rate is high.

Chronic gastritis

This condition may be either atrophic or hypertrophic. In the former mild inflammatory changes in the mucosa over a number of years may lead to thinning and a reduction in the number of glands and the presence of occult blood in the stools. This condition may be associated with pernicious anaemia, cholecystitis, cirrhosis of the liver and pancreatitis, or may follow large doses of irradiation to the stomach or occur along the line of anastomosis following partial gastrectomy. In the hypertrophic type the mucosa appears a dull red colour, has stiff and prominent rugae, and multiple erosions may appear as shallow ulcers. The patient complains of dyspepsia, but improvement in both cases will occur after the taking of a careful, non-irritant diet and treatment of any underlying conditions.

Dyspepsia

In this condition the symptoms of gastritis are present without any definite changes having taken place in the gastric mucosa. Dyspepsia may be associated with the intake of food, or such diseases as those relating to the gall bladder, appendix, colon and in cardiac or renal failure. Examination should include a barium meal in order that a gastric ulcer should not be missed.

Nervous dyspepsia occurs in people who are subjected to psychological stress. This condition may be relieved by the administration of antacids and anticholinergic drugs, or if necessary psychological therapy. In any case it is essential that investigations have been undertaken to exclude any gastrointestinal disorders and thus confirm the diagnosis.

Anorexia nervosa

Anorexia nervosa usually occurs in young females and may have progressed from a rigid slimming plan. Strictly speaking it should not be included as there is no evidence of any organic or functional disorder of the gastrointestinal tract, but so frequently patients with symptoms are referred to a gastroenterologist for diagnosis. Food plays a major part in this patient's life, as there is a real desire for it, but this is well controlled, often to the point of thinking that eating is sinful. Extreme loss of weight occurs, also constipation and amenorrhoea, the pulse rate slows but the person remains actively restless. Examination of the blood chemistry shows normal values, except for possible reduction in the excretion of 17-ketosteroids. When investigating this condition it is important to exclude other wasting diseases. Treatment is shared with the psychiatrist and aimed at getting the patient into a suitable psychological state where they have a desire to eat which may be achieved by psychotherapy, administration of insulin to stimulate appetite or the use of chlorpromazine. Occasionally feeding by a continuous intragastric infusion is needed.

Peptic ulceration

This term is used to describe ulcers which result from irritation by gastric juice of the gastrointestinal mucosa at any level, hence they may occur in the oesophagus, stomach, duodenum, ileum, jejunum (Zollinger–Ellison syndrome, *see* page 78) and at the site of a gastroenterostomy stoma. This chapter deals only with ulcers occurring in the stomach and duodenum.

Duodenal ulcers are about three times more common than gastric ulcers, and in the former these occur in a ratio of 4:1, male:female, as opposed to roughly equal incidence in gastric ulcers. Persons belonging to the lower social classes tend to acquire gastric ulcers more frequently, whereas duodenal ulcers occur with roughly equal incidence amongst all social classes. People with blood group O would appear to be more susceptible to developing a duodenal ulcer, and certainly there is a familial tendency for both gastric and duodenal ulcers. A combination of factors predisposes to the incidence of peptic ulcers. These concern the environment, geographic areas, type of diet, smoking, alcohol and the prolonged administration of some drugs. The actual mucosa will also have an effect, together with the amount of acid secreted. In gastric ulceration there may be a reduction in the amount of acid produced, but this is associated with a decrease in acid resistance by the mucosa, whereas in duodenal ulcer there is an increase in gastric secretion which is not adequately offset by the buffering action of the mucus produced as well.

Diagnosis
History. The patient will probably complain of having experienced dyspepsia which may have lasted for weeks or months with periods of remission. Pain is often described as 'aching' or 'hunger' in type occurring in the upper epigastric region, and may be relieved by taking food. The patient with a gastric ulcer may find that pain starts about an hour after a meal and continues until the stomach empties when a period of relief occurs; whereas in duodenal ulceration the pain occurs two to three hours after a meal and is only relieved by the next meal. These latter patients tend to be woken during the night by pain, and in both cases patients will agree that their pain can be relieved by the taking of antacids or having a warm drink. In the chronic type of peptic ulceration pain features as the chief symptom but others may be present, such as nausea and vomiting, heartburn, acid regurgitation and effects on the appetite and colonic action. If attacks of pain are severe they may be accompanied by a feeling of nausea which may culminate in vomiting. Sometimes large quantities are vomited nine or ten hours after a meal; this is suggestive of pyloric stenosis or the formation of an hour-glass stomach where constriction has occurred as a result of scarring and fibrosis causing the stomach to become grossly overdistended, although in the latter instance vomiting may occur soon after a meal is taken. Heartburn is a common symptom and occurs as a retro-sternal pain, sometimes associated with the regurgitation of acid into the oesophagus and mouth. During a painful episode the patient may well not eat sufficiently and consequently weight loss will occur, but this weight may be regained during a period of remission. Often the older patient is afraid to eat and may therefore suffer from malnutrition. Spasticity of the colon may occur and patients complain of constipation, the abdominal discomfort associated with this being relieved by defaecation.

Examination. Examination of the patient will include a physical examination and certain diagnostic tests including barium X-ray, endoscopy and biopsy. Deep palpation of the epigastric region may cause the patient to experience a sharp pain over a localized area

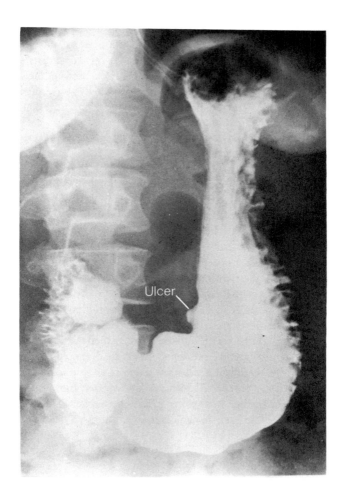

Fig. 18. *X-ray following barium meal showing gastric ulcer.*

where the actual ulcer is present. Peptic ulceration may exist alongside other diseases, and whilst making a general examination the doctor should not exclude other conditions. A barium meal will reveal the site of a gastric ulcer in the majority of cases, most commonly these are to be found on the lesser curvature of the stomach and show as a small niche filled with barium on the X-ray film. Ulcers occurring on the greater curvature are less frequent and tend to become malignant. The majority of duodenal ulcers occur in the first part of the duodenum; these cause an alteration in the contour of the duodenal cap due to the spasm and mucosal swelling which the ulcer has caused, which eventually may show as actual scarring. Duodenal ulcers never become malignant. Examination of the gastric and duodenal mucosa with the aid of a fibre-optic gastro- or duodenoscope, plus removal of a small portion of suspicious tissue will also prove an aid to diagnosis, especially if malignancy is suspected. Estimation of the level of acid secretion may be achieved by the use of the pentagastrin test, the procedure being the same as for a histamine test but a synthetic form of gastrin is injected. Normal levels of gastric secretion are found in gastric ulceration, a high level in duodenal and very high in the Zollinger–Ellison syndrome. Abnormally low levels occur in pernicious anaemia and carcinoma of the stomach. If a very high acid level is found, as this is indicative of the Zollinger–Ellison syndrome then the serum gastrin level should be estimated in order to facilitate diagnosis. Examination of the blood to reveal a possible anaemia should also be made, together with tests for occult blood in the stools; these investigations only point further to a lesion in the gastrointestinal tract, but will not indicate the area in which it is situated.

Treatment
Treatment of an uncomplicated gastric or duodenal ulcer takes account of several factors:

Rest in bed, preferably in hospital for two to three weeks. In this way the patient can often be removed from the various stressful situations which may aggravate the ulcer. Some doctors feel this is unnecessary if drugs which specifically encourage healing of the ulcer are employed, but there is some evidence to suggest that gastric ulcers heal more readily if the patient rests.

Diet should be as near normal as possible, ensuring that the patient has smaller, more frequent meals and avoids highly spiced and irritant foods. There is little necessity for giving puréed or sieved foods, and much to be gained from seeing that the patient has a well balanced nutritious diet, supplemented at intervals with a warm milk drink if pain occurs. Occasionally a continuous intragastric infusion of milk is ordered by the doctor in which one to two litres of milk are given over a twenty-four hour period. The observant nurse will note how much her patient eats and what foods are rejected, and will endeavour to make good the deficiency by offering something the patient would prefer.

Drugs. There are three main groups of drugs employed in the treatment of peptic ulceration: alkalis and antacids; anticholinergic and antispasmodic drugs; and specific drugs to encourage healing of the ulcer.

Alkalis and antacids. Sodium bicarbonate effectively neutralizes gastric juice, but some patients have developed an alkalosis with long term use. Aluminium hydroxide (dose 0·5–1 g orally) is an effective antacid and may be given either in tablet form or as a colloidal solution. Some magnesium salts are little absorbed by the intestine and therefore there is less danger of alkalosis, but because of their tendency to retain fluid they may cause diarrhoea. Magnesium trisilicate (dose 0·5–2 g orally) is a slow acting and effective antacid, without alkalosis and diarrhoea as side effects. Antacids in tablet form which can be sucked when pain commences are useful, i.e. Nulacin (whole milk, calcium and magnesium salts).

Anticholinergic and antispasmodic drugs are mainly related to atropine which inhibits the action of the vagus nerve, thus reducing gastric motility and secretion. Unfortunately it has other effects such as loss of visual accommodation and dryness of the mouth, retention of urine, constipation and tachycardia. Because of the side effects of the anticholinergic drugs they are unsuitable for patients with prostatic enlargement and acute glaucoma. A synthetic preparation such as propantheline bromide (Pro-Banthine, dose 15–30 mg orally before meals), is probably the most commonly used, and may be combined with phenobarbitone to give a sedative action as well.

Specific drugs are mainly carbenoxolone sodium (Biogastrone, dose 50–100 mg orally three times a day for three to four weeks), which aids the healing of gastric ulcers, and a similar preparation aimed to have maximum effect in the duodenum (Duogastrone). Carbenoxolone has the disadvantage of causing sodium retention which may result in oedema, hypertension and possibly congestive cardiac failure. It should therefore be given in association with a thiazide diuretic and additional potassium to counteract loss. Caved-S is a synthetic preparation from a similar liquorice base as carbenoxolone, but a substance from which the sodium retaining properties have been removed and therefore it does not give rise to electrolyte disturbances. Unfortunately this drug has not proved as effective as carbenoxolone in encouraging healing of the ulcer.

Smoking. Most physicians discourage patients with ulcers from smoking although there is no evidence to suggest that this actively encourages ulcer formation, but certainly the rate of healing of an existing chronic ulcer is increased in the absence of tobacco smoke. Other conditions which are common to this age group such as hypertension and peripheral vascular disease may also be improved if smoking is reduced.

Nursing care
The majority of patients admitted for this type of treatment for

peptic ulceration will find themselves in a medical ward. Some will resent admission to hospital and on comparison with some of their more ill companions in the ward will feel their stay in hospital is not justified. The nurse then has the sometimes difficult task of encouraging these patients to rest in bed, seeing that they are only up for toilet purposes if this is permitted and ensuring that all necessary treatments and observations are carried out for a patient who generally appears not to be very ill. If the patient is not permitted to take a bath then a daily bed bath should be given, with particular attention to pressure areas and the use of frequent mouthwashes. Stimulation of the appetite by attention to the content and appearance of meals is important, and the anticipation of pain and the administration of prompt relief in the form of the prescribed drugs will encourage the patient to be calm and cooperative towards his treatment. The nurse must be aware that serious complications can occur at any time and must be constantly observing the patient and be ready to act in an emergency. Patients being treated with carbenoxolone sodium should have their temperature, pulse and blood pressure recorded daily, together with a record of their urine output, and twice weekly weighing. As constipation may be a problem, suitable aperients will need to be given as necessary. The patient should be situated in a quiet area of the ward, with access to radio and television, and be allowed visitors. The nurse must find time to spend with this patient, and also encourage some form of diversional therapy even if only encouraging the use of the hospital library facilities.

Complications of peptic ulceration

The main complications of this condition are: haematemesis and melaena, perforation, pyloric stenosis, penetration and carcinoma.

Haematemesis and melaena

Brisk haemorrhage from the gastrointestinal tract may be observed as either haematemeis or melaena, but often bleeding is confined to continuous oozing which may only show as a positive result for the presence of occult blood in the stools in a patient with an iron deficiency anaemia. This latter feature is more common in patients with a gastric rather than duodenal ulcer. When haematemesis occurs the patient appears shocked, is sweating and collapsed, requiring urgent admission to hospital. Treatment is aimed at restoring the circulating blood volume at first by an intravenous infusion of dextrose saline, and when blood is available, by giving a transfusion. An injection of morphine 10–15 mg is usually given on admission, this has the effect of reducing peristalsis and therefore has a haemostatic as well as calming effect. The patient will need to be made comfortable in bed and encouraged to rest quietly. If shock is severe the foot of the bed should be elevated. Observations of temperature, pulse, respirations and blood pressure should be recorded hourly at least, all vomit measured and saved for inspection. Likewise any stools passed should be saved, and the amount of urine passed recorded and a specimen tested routinely. An assessment of the patient's colour, pain and general condition should be made. As vomiting may continue, a bowl, paper tissues and mouthwash should be near at hand. The patient will be frightened, but should be reassured by the calm manner of the nurse. The relative too will need an explanation and reassurance and to be kept informed of changes in the patient's condition or plan of treatment. Surgery may be indicated once the general condition of the patient has been improved, or if bleeding continues for forty-eight hours. If bleeding ceases then full investigations may be carried out and treatment continued in a conservative manner. Prior to operation an oesophageal tube size 14FG (7-8EG) should be passed so that the aspiration of blood clots may be possible. A Ryle's tube should not be used as the lumen is too narrow.

Perforation

Perforation is the commonest cause of death from peptic ulceration, and usually occurs with sudden onset following a meal, producing a major emergency. The sudden severe pain and abdominal rigidity are due to the escape of gastric contents into the peritoneal cavity, causing severe irritation of the peritoneum. At this stage the contents are sterile and so infection is not a problem. The patient is cold and clammy, feeling nauseated and may vomit, respirations are shallow in depth and the rate is increased, blood pressure is normal and the pulse rate normal or raised. Bowel sounds are not heard. About two or more hours later the pain eases and the patient looks and feels better, although the abdomen is still very rigid and the respirations shallow. General peritonitis occurs between six and twelve hours after perforation, bacterial invasion being responsible for the increasing abdominal distension (pain and rigidity are less), the rise in temperature and pulse rate, and a possible further rise in the respiratory rate. Treatment of the condition is by surgical means, a laparotomy is performed and the perforated area closed, and the peritoneal cavity drained. Prior to this it is usual to give morphine once a diagnosis has been made, and then to correct the fluid and electrolyte balance by the administration of intravenous fluids. A Ryle's tube is passed and the stomach contents aspirated at intervals. The nurse is responsible for preparing the patient for operation, checking that the consent for surgery has been signed, that the patient wears some form of identification, a urine specimen is obtained and tested for sugar and protein, the abdomen is shaved, and the premedication given when ordered. Checking for prostheses, jewellery and make-up, and dressing in an operation gown must also be included, and all the while the nurse is observing the condition of the patient and recording pulse rate and temperature as necessary. Broad spectrum antibiotics will probably be prescribed, and it must be appreciated that the risk of peritonitis occurring increases with each hour's delay following perforation. Postoperatively the patient will continue having intravenous fluids for thirty-six to forty-eight hours until bowel sounds are heard. Small quantities of fluid can then be taken by mouth, gradually increasing to a light and then full diet provided no vomiting or discomfort occurs. The Ryle's tube will have continued to be aspirated hourly until there is minimal aspirate and then it will have been removed. If a drainage tube is present draining the peritoneal cavity it will probably be shortened on the second and third post-operative days and removed when drainage is minimal. The dressing over the drainage tube may require changing at least twice a day, but that covering the abdominal incision should be disturbed only if necessary, and the sutures removed at about the eighth day. Drugs in the form of analgesics and aperients will have been given as necessary. Mobilization of the patient should be encouraged as soon as his condition permits, and the nurse should supervise active movements to prevent respiratory complications and deep vein thrombosis. Care should be taken of the patient's toilet needs, and this includes adequate mouth care and attention to pressure areas.

Pyloric stenosis

This usually occurs as a complication of a duodenal ulcer situated near the pylorus. The patient complains of distension associated with nausea following a meal and then the vomiting of large amounts. The attacks of severe pain which often occur are relieved by vomiting. Loss of weight, dehydration and signs of malnutrition will eventually be present. Diagnosis may be assisted by barium examination, and other investigations will show anaemia and electrolyte imbalance. Alkalosis may occur as a result of repeated vomiting, and a raised blood urea occurs due to the dehydration. The patient should be admitted to hospital in order that gastric aspiration can be carried out, the dehydration and electrolyte imbalance corrected and treatment for anaemia and malnutrition given prior to surgery. Antibiotics may be given as the stomach is likely to have become infected. Operation usually consists of a vagotomy and pyloroplasty to enable the stomach to empty effectively.

Penetration

When an ulcer situated on the posterior wall of the stomach continues to erode, it may penetrate into an adjacent organ such as the liver or pancreas without emptying the gastric contents into the peritoneal cavity. An exacerbation of symptoms occurs, with the pain increasing in severity and being felt in the back. Surgical treatment is usually indicated, although symptoms may subside with medical care.

Carcinoma

Malignant change occurs in about 6% of all gastric ulcers (never in duodenal) and presents difficulty in diagnosis as the majority do not produce any noticeable changes in the symptoms. Weight loss and anaemia continue, and mild jaundice may occur due to liver involvement. Surgery is usually indicated.

Surgical treatment

Surgical treatment for peptic ulceration may be undertaken for a number of reasons. These include: perforation, penetration, haemorrhage, pyloric obstruction, hour-glass contraction, malignancy and failure of the ulcer to heal when treated medically.

The first three indications are likely to necessitate emergency surgery, whereas the remainder may be done on a planned basis although a degree of urgency still exists.

Pre-operative care

The patient should be admitted several days prior to operation so that any outstanding investigations may be completed. Apart from the routine preparation for operation a patient about to undergo this type of surgery will require the abdomen to be shaved from the nipple line to the pubis, and minimal bowel preparation in the form of suppositories or disposable enema. Smoking should be discouraged, and a high protein diet with additional vitamins given. Treatment of anaemia may be carried out prior to operation, or blood be cross-matched and available for transfusion whilst surgery is taking place. The patient with pyloric stenosis will require a daily washout of the stomach using a large oesophageal tube attached to either a funnel or Senoran's evacuator. Most surgeons withhold food for twelve hours and permit fluids to within six hours of

operation; they also require a Ryle's tube to be passed immediately
pre-operatively.

Choice of operation
Partial gastrectomy is often the operation of choice, and this may
take several forms. The Billroth I technique performed for gastric
ulceration involves removal of the main ulcer bearing area (lesser
curvature), about half the greater curvature and consequently the

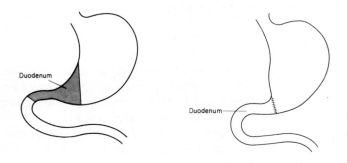

Fig. 19. *Before and after Billroth I operation (the shaded area is removed).*

whole of the pyloric antrum. The duodenum is then anastomosed to
the remainder of the stomach. The Billroth II or Polya gastrectomy
is suitable for removal of a duodenal ulcer. Here the pyloric antrum
of the stomach is removed leaving a larger area of the stomach than
in the previous operation, the jejunum is brought up and anastomosed to the stomach, whilst the detached duodenum forms a
blind loop.

Both these operations entail removal of a large part of the
secreting area of the stomach and therefore gastric acidity is considerably reduced. Vagotomy and pyloroplasty may be used effectively for both gastric and duodenal ulcers. Division of the vagus
nerves may be total or selective, the main objects being to reduce the

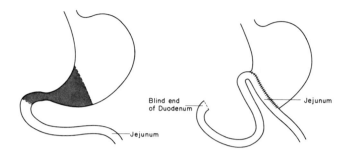

Fig. 20. *Before and after Polya operation (Billroth II), (the shaded area is removed).*

stimulation for the production of gastric juice and also reduce gastric motility. This operation does not remove the ulcer but induces an environment in which healing may take place. Vagotomy alone is unsatisfactory, due to the reduction in gastric motility, stasis of the stomach contents occurs and the patient will complain of a feeling of distension, vomiting and sometimes diarrhoea;

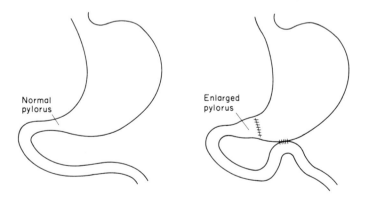

Fig. 21. *Before and after pyloroplasty and gastroenterostomy.*

consequently a drainage procedure must be part of the total operation. Pyloroplasty is often employed, whereby an incision is made in the pylorus, the divided edges being sutured at right angles to enlarge the pyloric opening. Alternatively, a gastroenterostomy may be done, where a loop of jejunum is anastomosed to the posterior surface of the pylorus thus forming a second exit from the stomach.

Complications following operations on the stomach

Complications which may arise soon after operation include haemorrhage from along the line of anastomosis, stomal obstruction due to oedema of the tissues surrounding the actual opening into the small gut, and duodenal fistulae caused by avascular necrosis occurring along the closed end of the blind loop of the duodenum.

The majority of the post-operative complications occur later and include:

Recurrence of ulceration. Further ulcers may form along the lines of anastomosis, or the original ulcer may fail to heal following vagotomy. Recurrence is related to the type of operation performed, about two per cent following Polya gastrectomy and a slightly higher rate after vagotomy and gastroenterostomy. Symptoms usually recur within two years. It may be necessary for a vagotomy to be performed if this has not already been undertaken, or the gastroenterostomy to be replaced by a partial gastrectomy.

Dumping syndrome. This term refers to the epigastric discomfort experienced by some patients within about half an hour of taking a meal. It is a complication likely to follow partial gastrectomy. The patient experiences nausea, sweating, tachycardia, feels faint and unsteady on the feet and may collapse. If vomiting occurs it usually relieves the symptoms, as does lying down. The blood sugar level rises during such an attack hence the condition is not due to hypoglycaemia. The condition is thought to be due to the sudden distension of the jejunum which causes an autonomic vasodilatation of the intestinal wall and a subsequent drop in the circulating plasma volume. With the patient in the recumbent position alterations in blood volume do not occur. Treatment is to suggest taking smaller meals and lying down for a while after eating. These symptoms are likely to be worse in the immediate post-operative period, but in time adjustment is made and recovery occurs within a few weeks or months.

Hypoglycaemic attacks occur after any type of gastric operation and affect about 5% of patients. The attacks come on about two to three hours after taking a meal, the patient experiencing giddiness, tremor, nausea and perspiration. There is a rapid rise in the blood sugar level by the sudden emptying of gastric contents into the duodenum, this is followed by a marked fall in the level over the next two hours. Hypoglycaemia is thought to be due to this. The attacks can be prevented by taking a small meal every two hours, but the patient should be reassured that over a period of time the attacks will become less frequent.

Nutritional disorders. Loss of weight may occur and is mainly due to the inability of the person to eat large meals. This is particularly so in the patient who has a heavy manual job and who may find it difficult to continue such work after operation. Malabsorption states may occur, giving rise to anaemia and steatorrhoea. Pernicious anaemia may not be evident for several years after a partial gastrectomy. About 5% of patients experience diarrhoea which may be episodic or persistent. The cause of this is not really understood, but attention to the diet may improve the condition. It is more likely to occur after vagotomy.

Pulmonary tuberculosis. Activation of an old pulmonary lesion may occur following gastric surgery, or a new case may occur. In the latter, recent partial gastrectomy features more frequently than other causes of new cases of tuberculosis. It is thought the reason an old

D

tuberculous lesion becomes active again or a primary infection occurs is due to the biochemical changes which take place in the body as a result of partial gastrectomy, and which produce a suitable tissue environment for the growth of the tubercle bacillus. Loss of weight may be another factor.

Post-operative nursing care
Care of the unconscious patient should be the prime consideration of the nurse, and the lateral position should be used until consciousness is regained and the patient can be sat up in bed well supported by pillows. The gastric contents may be aspirated intermittently at hourly intervals at first, progressing to two hourly on the second post-operative day. Some surgeons prefer the gastric tube to be attached to an electric pump so that continuous gentle suction can be maintained. The gastric tube is removed when the aspirate is minimal and the patient is taking fluids satisfactorily by mouth. Intravenous fluids will usually be given for the first twenty-four to forty-eight hours, using dextrose/saline and normal saline, giving an intake of three litres each day. Bowel sounds will probably be heard after thirty-six to forty-eight hours, when small measured quantities of fluid may be given frequently, the amount increasing until a light diet can be introduced. The patient may take a full diet as soon as he wishes. The wound may have a drainage device, either the Redivac type or a corrugated tube draining into a dressing. For the former the nurse must check the vacuum in the drainage container, and for the latter the tube will probably require shortening daily. In either case the tube will be removed about three days after operation when drainage ceases. Sutures may be removed from about the eighth day. If clips have been used these should be taken out twenty-four hours earlier. At first pain will need to be controlled by the injection of pethidine hydrochloride 50–100 mg four to six hourly, but on the day following operation mefenamic acid or pentazocine may provide adequate analgesia. The nurse must ensure that discomfort is relieved in order that the patient is able to cooperate with physiotherapy and mobilization which should start from the first post-operative day and be gradually increased. At first the nurse will

be required to give all toilet care to the patient paying particular attention to frequent oral hygiene. Observations of temperature, pulse and blood pressure should be recorded, together with the fluid intake and urinary output. At the end of about ten days the patient should be ready for discharge from hospital, the wound should be healed, the patient mobile and able to care for his own toilet needs, and be taking a full diet of smaller and more frequent meals. A period of convalescence should be encouraged before resuming work, and the patient asked to return for examination in about a month's time.

NEOPLASTIC CONDITIONS

Both benign and malignant tumours may be present in the stomach of which the latter are by far the most common.

Benign tumours

Benign tumours are mainly the adenomata which arise in the glandular parts of the epithelial tissue. These tumours may become pedunculated and are often called gastric polyps. They occur in patients with achlorhydria and atrophic gastritis, and are therefore often present in pernicious anaemia, where they are thought by many to be a premalignant condition; carcinoma of the stomach frequently occurs in this disease. Symptoms include epigastric pain, loss of weight and anorexia. Other benign tumours which may be present are the lipoma, fibroma and neuro-fibroma. In all cases treatment is by surgical resection of the tumour.

Malignant tumours

Malignant tumours include carcinoma and sarcoma, the former being the most common and accounting for many of the deaths each year in this country from malignant neoplasms. It is a condition which affects the middle aged and elderly male more frequently than the female. Incidence of carcinoma of the stomach shows a familial tendency, and is more often found in persons with Group A Rhesus positive blood. Environmental factors also play a part in the incidence of carcinoma, the mortality from this condition being much higher amongst the Japanese than the British. This factor has of course prompted research into the cause and various theories have been put forward which include differences in soil composition, occupations and social class. Twenty-five per cent of ulcers occur on the lesser curvature and fifty per cent in the pyloric antrum, hence there is considerable risk of an existing gastric ulcer eventually showing neoplastic changes.

Carcinoma of the stomach is of different types:

Adenocarcinoma
Malignant changes usually occur in an existing polyp and there is an increase in size.

Polypoid type

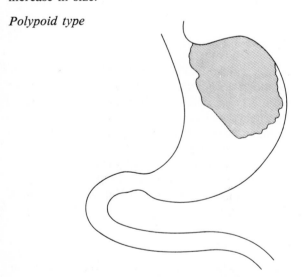

Fig. 22. *Polypoid tumour of stomach (the shaded area indicates tumour projecting into lumen of stomach from fundus).*

This is a soft, bulky growth which projects into the lumen of the stomach, but eventually invades the stomach wall and adjacent structures. This type readily produces metastases which infiltrate the nearby lymph nodes and the liver.

Malignant ulcer
The central part of this tumour appears ulcerated, with a raised and thickened surrounding edge. As with the polypoid type this readily metastasises, involving the liver and lymph nodes.

Linitis plastica
This tumour affects the entire stomach by infiltrating throughout the wall causing it to become thick and firm—often described as the 'leather bottle' stomach. This tumour may give rise to secondary growths, in women these are frequently to be found in the ovary (Krukenberg tumour). The patient with carcinoma of the stomach

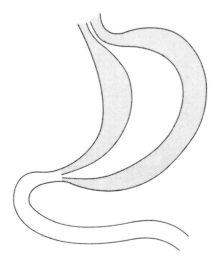

Fig. 23. *Linitis plastica (shading indicates gross thickening of stomach wall).*

may have few symptoms at first and these will vary, although the majority will experience some abdominal discomfort, weakness, weight loss and possibly dysphagia. Haematemesis, malaena and perforation may occur later. In some patients secondary deposits are found in the liver, bones and peritoneum before gastric disturbances occur and the primary tumour is located in the stomach. Examination of the patient may reveal an irregular, craggy mass on palpation of the abdomen, together with an enlarged liver. Barium meal X-ray will often show a filling defect in the stomach as the lumen is reduced by the presence of the tumour. Cytological examination may be necessary, and a biopsy should be carried out with the aid of a fibre-optic gastroscope.

Prognosis for this condition is poor, but irrespective of treatment a proportion of patients survive five years.

Treatment and nursing care

Less and less surgery is being performed for gastric carcinoma, and more use is being made of cytotoxic drugs such as methotrexate and cyclophosphamide. Radiotherapy has been shown to be of only limited value for this condition. An important aspect of nursing care is the relief of pain, which tends to become continuous and is unrelieved by taking alkalis. The nurse should use her discretion with regard to the time of giving analgesics and also the choice of drugs from those prescribed by the doctor, remembering that often a change in position, attention to the bladder or bowels, or a warm drink may make a less strong analgesic effective and therefore reduce the necessity of giving one of the Controlled Drugs. Nevertheless, the time will come when these are necessary and the nurse must be aware of her patient's needs and see that adequate analgesia is given.

Anorexia may present a problem to the nurse particularly as she will observe her patient to have lost weight and become thinner and more emaciated. No restrictions on diet should be made, and the patient should be encouraged to eat small quantities of whatever is fancied. Frequent drinks should be given and these may contain a high protein food such as Hycal. Jaundice may occur in the later stages, and skin irritation result due to the presence of bile salts in the subcutaneous tissues. A soothing application such as calamine lotion may be necessary. The patient should be encouraged to be ambulant, but as weakness progresses the nurse will need to assist or undertake aspects of personal care such as bathing. The patient may be nursed on a ripple mattress or similar bed to relieve pressure and help prevent the formation of pressure sores. The presence of the carcinoma may induce vomiting, which will be distressing to the patient who will need constant attention to be kept feeling and looking clean and fresh. The psychological problems associated with this condition must be anticipated by the nurse, and she should support the patient who may be well aware of the diagnosis and not want to die. An understanding nurse can help her patient through the stages of aggression and depression to a calm acceptance of the inevitable by her being with the patient, quietly answering questions and giving encouragement. The relatives also must be brought into this atmosphere of care and support, for they too may need guidance on how to talk to the patient and how they can help care for his physical needs.

CHAPTER 5

The Liver

The liver is the largest organ in the body weighing between 1200 and 1500 g in the adult, this being about one-fiftieth of the total body weight. In the baby the liver is even heavier in relation to the body weight due to the larger left lobe which undergoes a degree of atrophy after birth with the closure of the ductus venosus.

Development and structure

The liver starts its development along with that of the duodenum by the formation of a thickened area of the foregut into which a capillary plexus grows; this plexus originates partly from the umbilical vein, from whence the blood is conveyed to the heart. This structure forms a diverticulum, the apex of which divides into two solid buds, later to become the right and left lobes of the liver. Cylinders of cells grow into the vascular tissue of these buds, the cylinders constantly dividing and subdividing to form a spongy structure. In between the columns of cells will be found the vascular tissue, the origin of the liver sinusoids. At about the same time as the liver develops another solid bud arises from the foregut; this will become the gall bladder and occupy a position on the under surface of the liver. Canalization of the ducts occurs later, commencing from the liver. Although the liver is basically formed of two lobes it has two smaller lobes (these are really segments of the right lobe) to complete its structure, the quadrate lobe on the inferior surface and the caudate lobe on the posterior aspect. The right and left lobes are separated by a fold of peritoneum called the falciform ligament which passes from the umbilicus to the liver to the right of the midline and carries the ligamentum teres in its free border. The ligamentum teres is an obliterated remnant of the umbilical vein, the fetal blood vessel which conveyed oxygenated blood from the placenta through the umbilical cord to the liver. Shortly after birth it fibroses and

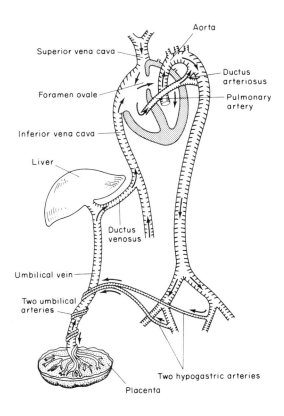

Fig. 24. *Fetal circulation.*

becomes a supporting ligament of the liver; some small veins accompany it and connect the left branch of the portal vein to other veins at the umbilicus. If obstruction occurs in the liver these veins surrounding the umbilicus are likely to become distended and prominent. Posteriorly the right and left lobes are separated by a fissure through which passes the ligamentum venosum which is a fibrous remnant of the ductus venosus, the fetal vessel which shunted blood from the umbilical vein to the inferior vena cava as it by-passed the liver. Another fissure on the inferior surface of the right lobe forms the porta hepatis, and through this the main blood vessels pass as they enter and leave the liver together with the common hepatic duct. The liver has a double blood supply, the portal vein which drains the intestines and spleen, and the hepatic artery which is one of the branches of the coeliac axis; immediately after entering the liver these vessels divide into branches which pass to both the right and left lobes. All venous blood from the liver drains into the right and left hepatic veins which empty directly into the inferior vena cava after leaving the liver; this latter makes a deep groove on the back of the liver as it passes up towards the thorax. Lymph drainage is to two groups of nodes, one group situated around the porta hepatis and the other in the mediastinum, the

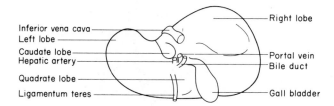

Fig. 25. *Inferior surface of the liver.*

lymph having been conveyed through an opening in the diaphragm. Nervous control of the liver is through the autonomic system, both sympathetic and parasympathetic fibres play a part. The nerves accompany the main blood vessels in through the porta hepatis and follow their branches right into the main liver tissue. The liver is almost entirely covered with peritoneum except for three areas: (1) where the liver is in direct contact with the diaphragm, which is known as the bare area of the liver; (2) the fossa through which passes the inferior vena cava; and (3) the fossa which carries the gall bladder.

The microscopic structure of the liver shows it to be made up of lobules, each containing a number of liver units, that is a central hepatic vein surrounded by liver cells which radiate out from the centre. At intervals are found the portal tracts which consist of the capillaries of the portal vein and the hepatic artery, together with a small bile duct. Blood passes from the capillaries on the perimeter of the liver unit along the sinusoids between the columns of liver cells into the central hepatic vein; the bile which is produced flows in the reverse direction between the liver cells (the bile pathways alternating with the blood sinusoids) towards the portal tract from where it passes to the bile duct.

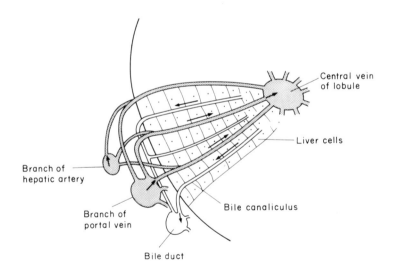

Fig. 26. *Part of the liver lobule.*

About 60% of the liver is made up of hepatic cells and it has been shown that cells present in different zones of the liver will perform a separate function. The walls of the sinusoids are lined by endothelial cells and at intervals will be found the Kupffer cells. These phagocytic cells are part of the reticulo–endothelial system and are concerned with the production of immune bodies and the removal of worn out red cells and other cell debris from the blood as it passes.

Examination and investigation of the liver

Examination of the liver may be considered under the following headings:

Palpation
The normal liver in the adult may be palpated along its lower border (which passes from the right tenth rib to just below the left nipple) when it moves in a downward direction for 1–3 cm on deep

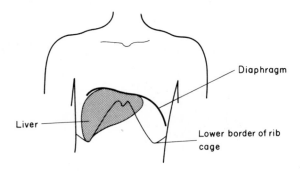

Fig. 27. *Surface markings of the liver.*

inspiration. Changes in size of the liver make it more readily palpable and this is likely to occur in such conditions as Hodgkin's disease, leukaemia, congestive cardiac failure and when metastases are present. Pulsation in the liver may be felt by the examining hands, one placed posteriorly and the other anteriorly, and this suggests incompetence in the tricuspid valve.

Percussion
Alteration in density will be observed during percussion over the liver; by this method the outline of the liver shape can be estimated.

Auscultation
In portal hypertension a venous hum may be heard, whereas an arterial murmur may suggest a hepatic tumour.

Radiology
A plain X-ray of the abdomen will show the size and shape of the liver and will help the doctor to decide whether the palpable liver is due to enlargement or displacement.

Radioactive scanning
One of three isotopes may be used to determine the size and function of the liver: (1) gold-198 (^{198}Au) is taken up by the Kupffer cells and outlines the liver; (2) iodine-131 (^{131}I) labelled Rose Bengal is taken up by the liver cells. This isotope does not give such a clear outline as when Au is used; and (3) technetium-99M (^{99m}Tc) gives a clear scan.

If lesions are present in the liver then these do not take up the isotope and will show as filling defects. A generalized decrease in uptake is suggestive of cirrhosis. Special preparation of the patient and after-care is necessary when these investigations are performed; details are to be found in Chapter 14.

Tests of liver function
These tests may be carried out on blood, urine and the faeces, for in this way the level of substances manufactured by the liver can be estimated as well as those either excreted or modified by the liver.

Tests on the blood
  Serum proteins. The liver manufactures albumin, fibrinogen,

prothrombin and transferrin amongst other proteins, normally the total being 60–80 g/l (6–8 g/100 ml) blood. By the use of radioactive isotopes the quantity present of the individual proteins can be measured, and variations from the normal values will give an indication to the diagnosis. For instance, the serum albumin level falls in cases of malnutrition, fever and chronic liver disease.

Serum bilirubin. Bilirubin is formed from haem following the breakdown of the red blood cell; this takes place in the spleen after a life of about one hundred and twenty days. Bilirubin is insoluble in water, and needs to be conjugated by the liver in order that it can be excreted either in the urine as urobilinogen or by the faeces as stercobilinogen. Bilirubin is carried to the liver attached to the plasma albumin, and is then acted on by glucuronic acid (conjugated) which converts it to the water soluble bilirubinogen. This passes to the gut as a constituent of bile where it is acted on by the

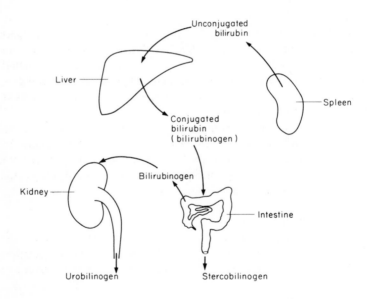

Fig. 28. *Bilirubin pathway.*

intestinal bacteria to form stercobilinogen and excreted in the stools. Some bilirubinogen is reabsorbed and conveyed to the kidney and subsequently excreted in the urine as urobilinogen. Unconjugated bilirubin remains as a fat soluble substance and when present in the subcutaneous tissues gives the characteristic yellow appearance of jaundice. The Van den Bergh test is the most usual one employed to estimate the total serum bilirubin present. The results of this test are given as 'indirect' or 'direct' bilirubin, which refer to unconjugated and conjugated bilirubin respectively. Normal serum contains $3 \cdot 4 - 13 \cdot 6$ µmol/l ($0 \cdot 2 - 0 \cdot 8$ mg/100 ml); this level will be raised in all forms of jaundice as a serum bilirubin level of over 34 µmol/l (2 mg/100 ml) corresponds with visible jaundice.

Serum enzymes. Alkaline phosphatase is excreted by the liver cells and the normal level is 3–13 King–Armstrong units/100 ml blood. This level will be raised in hepatic jaundice and where a tumour is present in the liver. The serum transaminases are enzymes normally present in the liver which are concerned with the synthesis of amino acids. Glutamic oxaloacetic transaminase (GOT) is also present in large quantities in the heart and skeletal muscles. If cell damage occurs this enzyme is released and will cause a marked increase above normal (5–17 I.U./100 ml blood); this situation is found in hepatic necrosis and in myocardial infarction. Glutamic pyruvic transaminase (GPT) is also present in liver, but less is found in heart and skeletal muscle. Therefore an increase in the serum level above normal (4–13 I.U./100 ml blood) is more significant of liver damage than the SGOT estimation. Other enzymes which may be estimated in the serum include lactic dehydrogenase, choline esterase and xanthine oxidase. Alteration in their amount will give some indication of liver damage.

Tests on the urine

Urobilin. In normal circumstances, only a very small amount of bilirubinogen is absorbed by the gut. It passes through the liver where no further action is taken and eventually finds its way to the kidney where it undergoes change to urobilinogen and is excreted in the urine, later being oxidized to urobilin. The total amount excreted in this way each day is very small, varying with the time at which a specimen of urine may be obtained for testing, but a marked increase in urobilin is suggestive of some pathological condition; the level may be increased suggesting hepatic cell damage as in cirrhosis, malignancy of the liver and virus hepatitis. Schlesinger's test may be used in which equal quantities of urine and a saturated solution of zinc acetate in absolute alcohol are placed in a centrifuge tube and one drop of tincture of iodine is added to change the urobilinogen to urobilin. The tube is centrifuged and a positive result is shown by a green fluorescence where the zinc has combined with urobilin. In normal urine this does not occur.

Bilirubin. Conjugated bilirubin may be excreted in the urine but is not normally present. In cases of jaundice due to liver cell damage or obstruction then a small amount of bilirubin may be found in the urine; the Ictotest may be used for this. In haemolytic jaundice the urine appears dark in colour, but this is due to urobilinogen. Only if the haemolysis is proceeding rapidly may a small amount of bilirubin be present in urine.

Tests on the faeces

Colour. Normal stools are dark brown in colour, but if complete biliary obstruction is present then the faeces will be pale. In hepatic jaundice the stools are either pale or normal in colour, whereas in haemolytic jaundice they are normal or dark.

Stercobilinogen. The amount of stercobilinogen present in the stools may be assessed but as this entails a lengthy process it is not often undertaken. It must be remembered that the normal bacteria of the gut convert conjugated bilirubin to stercobilinogen and therefore antibiotics should not be given when the stools are being collected for this investigation. There will be more stercobilinogen present when haemolysis and jaundice increase.

Needle biopsy of the liver

The decision to carry out this investigation must be made after due consideration of the patient's condition and the benefit that is likely to be gained, for the introduction of a needle into the liver carries a considerable risk to the patient. If the liver capsule is torn this could lead to a large haemorrhage and may prove fatal, similarly haemorrhage may occur in the patient who is already jaundiced. As a precaution all patients should have the prothrombin time estimated prior to this investigation and there should be one unit of blood cross-matched and available for use; if jaundice is present then the patient should receive 10 mg vitamin K daily for three days prior to biopsy. Sodium amytal 200 mg may be given thirty minutes before the procedure is carried out.

Technique. The patient lies supine with the right side near to the edge of the bed, and the right arm behind the head. A pillow placed under the left side will tilt the body slightly to the right. The patient turns the head to the left. The skin is cleaned, a local anaesthetic given and a small skin nick made with the scalpel. The intercostal approach is used, that is the eighth, ninth or tenth intercostal space in the mid-axillary line. Various needles are available but many

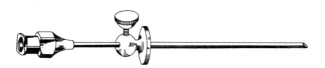

Fig. 29. *Menghini needle.*

prefer to use the Menghini needle. A syringe is filled with 3 ml of sterile saline, which is attached to the biopsy needle before it is inserted along the anaesthetized track into the subcutaneous tissues. Saline 1 ml is injected to clear the needle of any debris, and whilst the patient holds his breath on expiration the needle is quickly introduced through the intercostal space into the liver; expiration is maintained and the needle is quickly withdrawn. The tip of the biopsy needle is now placed under saline in a suitable receptacle, and a small amount of the saline in the syringe is injected in order to free the specimen from the needle. A small dressing may be placed over the biopsy site which may bleed for up to a minute from the puncture wound. If serious haemorrhage occurs bleeding is usually into the peritoneal cavity. The patient's pulse rate should be taken and recorded hourly for twenty-four hours, during which time the patient should remain in bed. An analgesic may be required for discomfort.

Liver biopsy may be carried out to determine the nature of a lesion shown up by a radioactive scan, for the diagnosis of malignant hepatic tumours, cirrhosis, cholestatic jaundice, and where granulomata are present in the liver and suggest sarcoidosis or tuberculosis.

It will be appreciated that for any one patient only a selection of these investigations will be carried out when assessing liver function in order to make a diagnosis; and that the history of the condition together with the findings of a physical examination are all part of the total investigation which should be made.

CONGENITAL AND ANATOMICAL ANOMALIES

Congenital anomalies occurring in the liver are few and may not give rise to symptoms but only be diagnosed at operation for some quite unrelated condition. They include:

(1) Accessory lobes. Only if the lobe twists on itself will this need to be corrected by surgery. Sometimes a projection of the right lobe of the liver extends down in to the right iliac fossa which is known as Reidel's lobe, but is not a true accessory lobe. It usually does not give rise to symptoms and therefore no treatment is necessary.

(2) Cough furrows. Parallel grooves may be seen on the convex surface of the right lobe of the liver passing in an antero-posterior direction. The furrows are formed by hypertrophied, diaphragmatic muscle bundles which exert pressure on the liver substance usually in association with a chronic cough. They are more common in women.

(3) Atrophy of the left lobe. This is caused by interference with the left branch of the portal vein. It may be present at birth when the left lobe loses its blood supply from the ductus venosus which becomes obliterated, the lobe undergoing degenerative changes which may persist into adult life; or it may occur later due to obstruction of the blood supply by the presence of malignant deposits or compression of the vessels.

TRAUMA

Rupture of the liver may result from a birth injury (breech delivery), during an epileptic fit or whilst surgery is being carried out, or most frequently as one among several injuries sustained in a road accident. Surgical treatment should be given as soon as possible. For a penetrating wound of the liver, drainage of the area is all that will be required. For a moderate tear, repair using catgut is necessary, whilst an extensive laceration will require some form of hepatic resection, probably a lobectomy. In this latter condition the common bile duct should be drained by a T-tube. Rupture of the liver still carries a considerable mortality (11·2%) but this has been very much reduced since the introduction of more modern surgical techniques.

JAUNDICE

This term is used to describe the yellow discolouration due to bilirubin becoming attached to the elastic tissue of the skin. When the plasma bilirubin level reaches 34 μmol/l (2 mg% (100 ml)) then jaundice is clinically apparent, but the staining remains for several days following a return to a normal serum bilirubin level. In jaundice bilirubin may be found in body fluids which do not normally contain it, such as the cerebrospinal fluid, milk, urine, semen and sweat.

Bilirubin undergoes a series of changes from the time it is

produced in the spleen until it is finally excreted from the body, and anywhere along this pathway (Fig. 28) the process may be interfered with and give rise to jaundice. Classification of the types of jaundice is therefore related to factors which effect these changes along the route, but it is important to note all the relevant clinical signs that are present in order that a correct differential diagnosis can be made.

Types of jaundice

Haemolytic jaundice

Excess haemolysis of red blood cells causes an increased production of bilirubin which is likely to remain unconjugated. It may be congenital or acquired. Bilirubin is excreted in the stools which are dark in colour, but little or no bilirubin is present in the urine. The skin has a lemon yellow tint due to both the jaundice and anaemia which results from the reduction in number of healthy red cells. Diagnosis may be assisted by tests to measure red cell fragility, or the presence of antibodies (Coombs test) and also the number of reticulocytes present. The life span of the red cells can be measured by labelling them with radioactive chromium.

Due to failure to conjugate bilirubin

Inability of the liver to conjugate bilirubin may be due to its immaturity such as may be found in the premature baby. Until the fetus is born the excretion of bilirubin is undertaken by the mother, but immediately following birth the baby must do this for himself. The task is even more difficult if he is born very prematurely and has not the full complement of the necessary enzymes. Failure to conjugate bilirubin along with inability on the part of the liver cells to transport and excrete bilirubin is a feature of a congenital condition of hyperbilirubinaemia which is found in young people who have a long history of jaundice. It is a condition which tends to be familial. Liver function tests may prove normal but there is a raised plasma bilirubin level.

Due to diffuse hepato-cellular damage

Where liver cells are damaged as in acute and chronic hepatitis then large amounts of conjugated bilirubin may be present in the blood.

Cholestatic jaundice (intrahepatic)

The term cholestatic refers to obstruction to the bile pathway anywhere along its route from the liver cell to the duodenum. Intrahepatic causes are mainly due to obstruction in the bile canaliculi caused by drug sensitivity or acute virus hepatitis, although other factors may be responsible. These types of jaundice are of rapid onset with pyrexia, slight weight loss and pruritus. Slight enlargement of the liver may be present and urobilinogen appears later in the urine; the stools are mainly pale in colour. Carcinoma of the liver and biliary cirrhosis are two other causes of this condition. In carcinoma the liver is enlarged and irregular in shape and there is other evidence of underlying disease; whereas in cirrhosis the biochemical tests of liver function are abnormal, and other features such as ascites and spider naevi may be present.

Cholestatic jaundice (extrahepatic)

This is often referred to as obstructive jaundice. This mechanical obstruction is outside the liver and may be due to something blocking the bile bathway such as a gall stone in the common bile duct (see Chapter 6) or a carcinoma of the head of pancreas (see Chapter 7) which presses on the bile duct particularly at its entrance to the duodenum. In obstruction due to gall stones the patient is usually an obese female aged about forty years complaining of biliary colic and pruritus. Rigors are common. Rarely occult blood may be present in the stools which are intermittently pale in colour. Urobilinogen is present in the urine. In carcinoma of the head of the pancreas the patient is often over fifty years, deeply jaundiced with constant epigastric pain and pruritus. The liver is enlarged and there is lack of bilirubin in both the stools and urine. The serum bilirubin level shows a steady rise. The temperature is usually normal.

In view of the many factors responsible for jaundice it is necessary that as much information as possible be obtained from the patient as to the history of the condition. This should include the occupation of the patient, family history, any previous conditions treated by drugs and whether the patient has been in contact with other jaundiced persons.

Jaundice in the newborn

Because of the low oxygen tension present in the blood in the placenta where exchange of gases takes place between the maternal and fetal blood supplies the fetus has been equipped with a higher ratio of red blood cells ($6-7 \times 10^{12}/l$ of blood) than will be needed after birth; to take up a greater quantity of oxygen. During the first few days of life the baby haemolyses some of these unwanted red cells and attempts to conjugate and remove the excess bilirubin and in so doing the normal healthy infant born at term may exhibit a mild degree of physiological jaundice usually on the second or third day of life. By giving the baby an adequate amount of fluid (water is suitable, it does not need to be a milk feed) the degree of jaundice may be minimal and has usually faded by the eighth day. The jaundice is often more severe in premature infants or where there is haemolytic disease of the newborn (due to blood group or Rhesus incompatibility) and in babies suffering from severe infection. In these situations the liver is overwhelmed by the amount of bilirubin for conjugation and can only deal with a proportion of it, hence large quantities of unconjugated bilirubin (fat soluble) are in circulation in the blood and may become attached to the basal ganglia and brain stem nuclei giving rise to the condition of kernicterus. Kernicterus is characterized by fever, meningism and convulsions which may lead to death, or if recovery occurs there may be mental retardation, deafness, cerebral palsy or athetosis. Kernicterus may also result from the administration of salicylates and sulphonamides. For the baby that appears more than mildly jaundiced, blood should be taken for estimation of the serum bilirubin level, importance being placed on the ratio of conjugated to unconjugated bilirubin present. As the jaundice increases, further blood specimens should be taken and a graph plotted of the rise in the bilirubin level against hours of life. It is the continuous rise in the bilirubin level which is significant and if this curve rises sharply then kernicterus may result. The paediatrician will decide what is the safe maximum level the serum bilirubin should reach before a replacement transfusion will be necessary for the baby; this may be at 255 μmol/l (15 mg/100ml). This treatment is carried out irrespective of the cause of the jaundice, and takes the form of introducing a cannula into a vein (preferably the umbilical vein if this is still patent) and by using a three-way connection removing about 10 ml of blood and replacing it with an equal quantity of fresh compatible blood. The procedure is repeated until about 80% of the baby's blood has been replaced, calculated on 160–200 ml/kg of body weight at birth. Once a replacement transfusion has been carried out observation of the depth of jaundice gives no indication of the serum bilirubin level, as the tissues take several days to revert to a normal colour. Therefore blood tests should be repeated daily until it is evident that the situation has been resolved. If the bilirubin level continues to rise it may be necessary to repeat the replacement transfusion.

Some babies remain jaundiced long after the time that physiological jaundice normally disappears. In the event that all blood tests prove to be normal it is worth considering the possibility that the baby may lack thyroid hormone and investigations to this effect should be carried out.

Jaundice occurring after one week of life

Some infants do not show signs of jaundice for several days or weeks and therefore the diagnosis cannot be physiological jaundice, but the condition may be due to one of the following:

Defective conjugation

This is a familial condition due to lack of conjugating enzymes present in the liver. Kernicterus may result and there is a high mortality rate.

Primary hepatitis

There is usually no evidence of blood incompatability and the cause may be unknown. Siblings may be affected. If the jaundice persists for three weeks then kernicterus may occur, also cirrhosis of the liver is a possible outcome. Occasionally hepatitis at this stage in life is due to congenital syphilis, galactosaemia and toxoplasmosis.

Obstructive jaundice

This may be due to some congenital abnormality of the biliary apparatus, usually atresia of the bile ducts (*see* Chapter 6). Investigation and treatment of the underlying cause where appropriate should be given. Also observation of the degree of jaundice and possible replacement transfusion carried out if the serum bilirubin has reached a critically high level.

INFECTIVE CONDITIONS OF THE LIVER

Liver abscess

Infection in the liver usually spreads along the bile ducts in the lobules and may give rise to a solitary abscess surrounded by fibrous tissue or multiple yellow abscesses about one centimetre in diameter; pus and small blood clots are likely to be present. The infection is usually of a mixed type, the predominating organism being the *Escherichia coli*, and staphylococcus, *Streptococcus faecalis* and *Clostridium welchii* may all be responsible. Liver abscess may be due to a number of causes these include:

(1) Secondary to existing infection such as acute appendicitis (more common in young people), infection in the gall bladder and diverticulitis.

(2) Secondary to obstruction of the biliary apparatus such as by a gall stone, carcinoma or stricture (more common in the older age group).

(3) Infection entering through the umbilical vein in the newborn, which may follow umbilical sepsis.

(4) Infection entering along the pathway of a penetrating wound of the liver.

(5) Unknown aetiology.

The patient may complain of a dull ache in the right hypochondrium which may radiate towards the right shoulder; there will be weakness and sweating. The patient looks toxic and wasted and the rise in temperature may be accompanied by rigors; both jaundice and anaemia may be present. On palpation the liver is enlarged and tender. Diagnosis of the condition is assisted by a liver scan which will show the exact location of the abscess.

Treatment

This is primarily by prevention of abscess formation by the early treatment of all acute abdominal infections. When an abscess becomes localized it should be drained surgically, and the patient given systemic antibiotics such as cephaloridine, kanamycin, ampicillin or cloxacillin depending on the sensitivity of the causative organism. If obstruction in the common bile duct predisposed to the formation of the abscess then this should be relieved when the acute condition has subsided. Death from liver abscess is still a possible outcome, or if recovery occurs then portal hypertension may result from a thrombus in the portal vein. This complication may require surgical treatment.

Virus hepatitis

Hepatitis is an acute inflammatory condition affecting the entire liver leading to cell necrosis. As the inflammation subsides regeneration of the liver cells takes place from the edge of the lobules towards the central vein. Other organs may become involved in this inflammatory reaction and these include the stomach, duodenum, jejunum, pancreas and kidney; the regional lymph nodes are likely to be enlarged. Two viruses are mainly responsible for hepatitis giving rise to two clinical conditions although there are similarities as to pathology and the course of the actual diseases.

Infectious hepatitis

The virus responsible for this is present in urine, faeces and droplets from the nose and pharynx, and can also be spread by transfusion of infected blood. The hepatitis may only be mild, but is likely to occur in epidemics amongst children and young adults, especially if the spread is by faecal contamination of water or food. Infectious hepatitis may have a short incubation period of only fifteen days and jaundice may or may not be present later. The Australia antigen is not found in the patient's serum.

Serum hepatitis

This type of hepatitis has a long incubation period of at least fifty days and maybe one hundred and sixty days, the virus being acquired mainly from infected blood or its products. In some cases spread occurs through urine, faeces and the oral route. It is likely to produce a severe inflammation affecting any age group, although cases are more likely to be sporadic. As with infectious hepatitis jaundice may or may not occur, and the blood may remain infective for several years after the initial attack. The Australia antigen is usually present in the serum within twelve days of the onset of symptoms and may remain for two to three weeks. This antigen may be found in the blood of otherwise healthy persons with no symptoms of the disease, yet they are capable of transmitting hepatitis.

In both infectious and serum hepatitis the spread of the condition may be by the needles, tubing, syringes and bottles used for giving all types of injections if these have been inadequately sterilized. These are conditions which may be spread by the communal use of equipment amongst those who are drug dependent, and may also occur from accidental inoculation of hospital and laboratory staff who are concerned with either the care of patients or their blood specimens. Hepatitis is an ever present risk to both patients and staff in a haemodialysis unit.

Clinical features

In both types of hepatitis the patient may complain of loss of appetite especially for fatty foods, and also have no wish to smoke or drink alcohol. Nausea, vomiting and abdominal distension may be present, and this contributes to the general malaise. The patient may experience pain under the right costal margin especially when lying on the right side. Pyrexia may be present but the rise in temperature is not sufficient to cause rigors, and there is a return to normal when the jaundice appears. Occasionally the patient experiences severe headache, also an urticarial rash may develop; this is more likely in serum hepatitis. Prior to the onset of jaundice the urine becomes darker in colour and the stools paler; blood tests will show a rise in the serum transaminase level, and if the course of the hepatitis is prolonged the serum albumin level falls. Within a few days of the onset of jaundice there is a start made towards a return to normal, and the patient enters the convalescent stage. In adults the illness usually lasts between two and six weeks. If jaundice does not develop then the same symptoms are present but the course of the disease is less severe and of a shorter duration.

Following recovery some patients fail to regain lost weight, suffer from anorexia and abdominal discomfort and naturally becomes anxious about their condition. Full investigations should be carried out: the results are likely to be normal and the patient should be told this and reassured that gradual improvement should be maintained but that it may be as long as one year before they feel really fit. The mortality rate is between one and two per thousand cases, probably more dying from hepatitis of blood-borne origin.

Prevention of hepatitis

In infectious hepatitis where spread is more likely by contact with human excreta, attention to sanitation, water supplies and personal hygiene is important and bed linen used by the patient should pass through an adequate laundering process. Gamma globulin may be given to high risk individuals such as pregnant women and close contacts of the patient, but this protection only lasts for about six months.

In serum hepatitis prevention should be directed towards adequate sterilization and care in the use of all equipment for taking and transfusing blood. All would-be blood donors should have their blood tested for the presence of Australia antigen, and those blood donors who come into contact with hepatitis should discontinue giving blood. All patients and staff in haemodialysis units should be similarly investigated at regular intervals; also patients attending leukaemia clinics. Gamma globulin offers no protection to this type of hepatitis.

Treatment and nursing care

The patient should be in a single room with full isolation precautions. Bed rest should be encouraged until the patient is free of symptoms and there is no jaundice and the liver is no longer tender on palpation. The patient should be offered a low fat diet, purely because this is more palatable, and when the appetite improves then high protein meals should be given. In severe cases where there is a possibility of hepatic coma developing the protein content of the diet should not be increased. Because of the risk of spread of infection the nursing staff should wear gowns, masks and disposable gloves while attending to the patient, and all bed linen should be conveyed separately to the laundry where it is passed through a disinfecting process. Disinfectant should be added to the urine and stools before their disposal; this may take the form of adding an equal volume of Sudol one per cent to the urine or covering the faeces with Sudol one per cent, both to be left for one hour. Disposable type crockery will be found useful. Apart from these measures both patient and staff must appreciate the importance of a strict hand-washing routine. Isolation nursing should be continued until the stools are no longer infective which is usually one week after the onset of jaundice. When the patient is fit enough to leave hospital he should be encouraged to take a long period of convalescence, avoiding exercise which proves tiring. A normal diet should be taken, but no alcohol for at least six months and preferably twelve. A follow-up appointment should be made for three months' time when the biochemical tests should be repeated.

INFLAMMATORY CONDITIONS

Cirrhosis

Cirrhosis is a condition likely to follow necrosis of liver cells and is characterized by the presence of fibrosis and nodules occurring in all parts of the liver. The fibrous tissue is arranged as bands of collagen fibres surrounding the nodules and joining them to the portal areas which causes disorganization of the actual liver structure; both fibrosis and nodules must be present, one alone does not constitute cirrhosis. The presence of nodules impedes the flow of blood through the liver substance eventually causing portal hypertension. To relieve this the sinusoids shunt blood from the portal zones to the hepatic vein and in so doing the blood by-passes functioning liver tissue and leads to vascular insufficiency. Cirrhosis may be caused by a number of factors, the two main ones being virus hepatitis and alcoholism; it may also develop in association with prolonged obstruction to the biliary pathway, cardiac failure, malnutrition, chemical poisons, galactosaemia, fibrocystic disease, congenital syphilis, as well as a large number of cases of unknown aetiology. Whatever the cause of cirrhosis two features will almost certainly be present, namely portal hypertension and inability on the part of the liver cells to carry out their normal functions. Cirrhosis does not affect the liver alone, but may be associated with other systems and conditions, these include:

(1) Malnutrition. Found frequently in those patients whose cirrhosis is due to alcoholism.

(2) Hepatic carcinoma (primary lesion). More frequent in cirrhosis following virus hepatitis.

(3) Abdominal hernia. Occurs as a complication of ascites.

(4) Spider naevi vascular changes in the skin. More likely to occur in the alcoholic patient.

(5) Renal failure. May be precipitated by the ascites or follow hypotension and shock.

(6) Eye signs may be present, such as lid retraction and colour blindness.

Patients with cirrhosis tend to have less systemic hypertension and atheroma and are consequently unlikely to have a myocardial infarction. Blood group A is a common genetic factor in persons developing cirrhosis.

Diagnosis

Not all patients with cirrhosis feel ill, but may deserve investigation of repeated epistaxis, indigestion and oedematous ankles. Biochemical tests should be carried out and these may prove normal or show a slight increase in the serum globulin and transaminase levels, associated with an excess of urobilinogen in the urine. These biochemical tests should be repeated at intervals in order to assess the progress of the condition. On abdominal palpation both the liver and spleen may be found to be enlarged, but occasionally the liver is contracted. Diagnosis is confirmed by taking a needle biopsy of the liver tissue, and scanning the liver using gold will reveal a patchy uptake of the isotope.

Prognosis

Once a diagnosis of cirrhosis has been made the course of the disease may be found to be slow and the patient dies eventually from another disease and not the hepatic condition. If cirrhosis progresses more quickly then liver failure may occur within months or years, and this will be associated with jaundice, ascites and hepatic coma; a full assessment of liver function at this stage is likely to show a prothrombin deficiency which is not due to lack of vitamin K, a low serum albumin and raised serum transaminase levels. Portal hypertension is very likely to develop and with this oesophageal varices which may bleed profusely. With adequate treatment of cirrhosis and the removal of some of the predisposing factors there is often a reasonable chance of the condition being arrested. Where cirrhosis is due to alcohol, if there is total abstinence then the chance of improvement is more favourable than for cirrhosis due to any other cause. If haemorrhage or infection precipitate cirrhosis and they are treated adequately then there is a better prognosis. This also applies to the response to treatment: if the condition shows signs of improvement within one month of commencing therapy then the outlook is more favourable.

For some patients the outcome is not so good, and features which indicate a poor prognosis include persistent jaundice, the development of neurological complications (although these may respond well to restrictions in dietary protein), ascites, persistent low prothrombin and albumin levels, and hypotension. Where haemorrhage complicates portal hypertension this may lead to coma and death.

Hepatic failure

Hepatic failure is mainly characterized by the presence of ascites and oedema; the former may be the first thing of which the patient complains along with jaundice. There is usually muscle wasting and weakness which contributes to the weight loss. Increased melanin in the skin causes more skin pigmentation, and the low platelet count will be responsible for the purpura seen on the arms, shoulders and shins. Spontaneous bruising and epistaxis occur as a result of the low prothrombin level. Clubbing of the fingers occurs and there is mild anaemia. There is a continuous mild pyrexia and a low blood pressure. Spider naevi, palmar erythema and white nails are all associated with this condition. The jaundice may deepen and this is an indication of poor liver cell function. Urobilinogen and stercobilinogen will be present in increased amounts in the urine and stool respectively.

Treatment of ascites and oedema

The formation of ascites and oedema can be partly controlled by the reduction in dietary sodium and the administration of diuretics. There was a time when ascites was treated by repeated paracentesis abdominis (drainage of ascitic fluid through a cannula introduced through the abdominal wall into the peritoneal cavity) but this procedure is not often employed now as it removes large amounts of body protein present in the fluid and does not deal with the cause of the fluid formation. Instead, a diuretic such as frusemide (Lasix)

40–80 mg orally daily is given along with a diet which allows less than 0·5 g sodium intake each day. The patient must be nursed in bed, and be weighed daily to assess response to treatment. Urine is collected over a twenty-four hour period to assess sodium output. In the diet an adequate amount of protein should be allowed (usually calculated as 1 g protein per kilogram body weight per day) but it is important to choose protein foods with a low sodium content, and this presents a problem for the dietician. Salt must not be used in cooking or added to meals.

Many protein foods which the patient might enjoy contain a high or medium sodium content, and the range of foods with little or no sodium is rather limited. Foods which may be eaten include:

Meat—beef, chicken, lamb, liver, rabbit, tongue (all contain medium amount of sodium and the quantity eaten should be strictly controlled).

Vegetables—broccoli, brussel sprouts, onions, lettuce, potatoes, tomatoes.

Fruit—oranges, apples, bananas.

Dairy foods—unsalted butter, cream.

Jams
Coffee
Sugar
Most cereal foods ⎫ all low sodium content

Fish has a high sodium content and should be avoided.

Portal hypertension

Portal hypertension is likely to be associated with enlargement of the spleen and the formation of oesophàgeal varices. During investigation of liver function the blood pressure in the portal vein should be measured by venography.

Treatment of bleeding oesophageal varices

As an emergency measure a Sengstaken tube may be passed (see Chapter 3) so that local pressure is exerted on the bleeding varices.

Blood should be made available for transfusion and vitamin K given intramuscularly. Vasopressin 20 units in 100 ml 5% dextrose may be given intravenously to lower the portal venous pressure; before this treatment is given an electrocardiogram should be recorded to check there is no evidence of coronary ischaemia as this is a contraindication to the use of vasopressin. The dose may be repeated in four hours, but if bleeding continues it is suggestive of liver failure. Occasionally emergency surgery in the form of a transoesophageal ligation of the varices is carried out through a thoracotomy incision, but a more satisfactory form of treatment is a portacaval anastomosis performed later when the bleeding has been controlled and the patient's condition improved. Whilst haemorrhage occurs the patient should receive a broad spectrum antibiotic such as neomycin, and the daily dietary protein intake should be reduced to about 20 g. In this situation it is possible that the patient develops signs of hepatic encephalopathy which may lead to pre-coma and coma, in which case all dietary protein should be withdrawn.

Portacaval anastomosis

The aim of this operation is to shunt the blood in the portal vein into the inferior vena cava and so reduce the portal venous pressure. Prior to operation the haemoglobin level must be restored, a course of a broad spectrum antibiotic commenced and the intake of dietary protein reduced for several days and entirely omitted for three days immediately prior to surgery.

There is a choice of two methods for this operation, either end-to-side anastomosis or side-to-side anastomosis. End-to-side anastomosis gives better results as there is a greater fall in the portal venous pressure and is the one usually undertaken. The portal vein is ligated and divided, the end conveying blood from the intestines is then anastomosed to the side of the inferior vena cava. The liver now receives its entire blood supply from the hepatic artery. In side-to-side anastomosis the portal vein is divided, one half is anastomosed to the inferior vena cava whilst the remainder continues its normal supply to the liver. When the success of the operation begins to be effective, it will be seen that the oesophageal varices and the distended collateral veins on the abdominal wall disappear, the spleen becomes smaller and the blood flow through the liver is

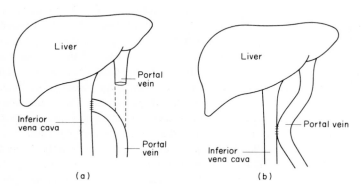

Fig. 30. *Portacaval anastomosis; (a) end-to-end anastomosis; (b) side-to-side anastomosis.*

reduced. Encephalopathy may result from the large amounts of nitrogenous matter present in the circulation which have not been through the liver for modification.

Alternative therapy for cirrhosis

Occasionally corticosteroids such as prednisolone have been used to treat cirrhosis, but on the whole this has not proved very successful. Immuno-suppressive drugs such as 6-mercaptopurine and azothioprine may be used for cirrhosis complicating virus hepatitis. The removal of toxic substances (particularly protein) from the blood may be carried out by exchange transfusion.

Hepatic pre-coma and coma

This condition may complicate any aspect of cirrhosis and subsequently lead to the death of the patient. As cell failure progresses liver functions become more impaired and the substances present in circulating blood are toxic to the brain. In liver disease the brain cells are particularly sensitive but would not be affected in a normal healthy state. Nitrogen in the diet passes straight into the systemic circulation because the liver is unable to deal with it. Also the intestinal bacteria act on the nitrogen content in the gut and produce a toxic substance; this latter problem can to a certain extent be overcome by reducing the intestinal flora by the use of a broad spectrum antibiotic. Failure of the liver to metabolize ammonia may also precipitate coma. Occasionally acute psychiatric states such as paranoid schizophrenia and hypomania occur several months after portacaval anastomosis due to cerebral intoxication.

Clinical features

There is a reduction in spontaneous movement and the patient becomes apathetic with a fixed stare and sleeps a lot. Personality changes are noted, childishness and irritability occur and there is intellectual deterioration. The speech becomes slurred and the voice monotonous. If an electroencephalogram is recorded there is slowing of the electrical waves. When the patient is asked to extend the arms, there is irregular flexion and extension of the fingers and wrists. This is known as 'flapping' tremor and is not specific to hepatic pre-coma but is found in other 'failures'—renal, cardiac and respiratory.

Treatment

All dietary protein should be discontinued and the patient given 6720 kJ (1600 calories) daily mainly of carbohydrate in the form of glucose. When improvement occurs then 20 g protein a day may be started, the diet being increased by this amount on alternate days. The response to treatment following an acute episode is usually good, and the patient quickly achieves a normal daily protein intake with no ill effects, but where the situation is more chronic then probably 40–60 g protein daily is the maximum that the liver can cope with adequately. During this time vitamins B and K should be given in the parenteral fluids, and antibiotics such as neomycin 6 g daily in divided doses should also be given. Besides reducing the protein intake treatment should include that of the predisposing factors, which may be haemorrhage, infection, alcoholism and electrolyte imbalance.

Nursing care in cirrhosis

In an acute phase the patient should be admitted to hospital for bed rest, dietary control and chemotherapy. The low sodium and low protein diet which may be ordered is likely to prove unpalatable to the patient and the nurse will need to give much encouragement to get the patient to eat. Difficulties may well arise with the patient whose cirrhosis is due to alcohol; when this is totally removed from the diet the patient may well become restless, uncooperative and aggressive. Diazepam is probably the safest drug to use to calm this patient; as the majority of drugs are detoxified by the liver the selection must be made with great care. The nurse will be responsible for making and recording observations on the patient, and these should include weighing daily, temperature, pulse and respiratory rates four hourly and also the blood pressure. The stools will need to be saved for occult blood estimation. The doctor will palpate the abdomen and examine the size of the liver each day, and request that the haemoglobin and electrolyte levels be estimated. There is a risk of pulmonary infection and also oedema; the nurse can help prevent these complications by keeping the patient sitting upright comfortably supported by backrest and pillows, and by encouraging deep breathing and the expectoration of sputum. The physiotherapist will also help the patient in this respect. A fluid balance chart should be maintained indicating all fluid taken by mouth or parenterally, and all fluid lost as urine or vomit. The patient may be thin due to malnutrition. Therefore the prevention of pressure sores is of utmost importance, and the use of such devices as sorbo rings, sheepskin pads and a ripple mattress should be considered. Where jaundice is present then skin irritation may cause a problem due to the presence of bile salts in the tissues; this may be relieved by the application of a soothing lotion such as calamine.

The care of the patient in hepatic coma will be primarily that of the unconscious person, and so the patient should be nursed in the lateral or semiprone position to ensure an adequate airway. The patient should be turned at two hourly intervals. All fluids will be given either intravenously or by the nasogastric route. It may be preferable to catheterize the patient and allow the bladder to drain continuously; catheter care and that of the urethral meatus is important and should be carried out at least twice daily.

Following recovery from an acute episode of cirrhosis the patient will need a period of convalescence during which time he must be helped to adjust to the restrictions which will be imposed on him; these may include those of diet (mainly sodium and protein) and also alcohol. To entirely abstain from alcohol may require great strength of character, and this may impose a tremendous strain on someone who because of their inadequacy or depression way back in the past took to drinking, and who may have failed several times to break the habit. Psychological help will be required, and the nurse must encourage the patient to accept this and so help him to see the benefit to his health if he refrains from alcohol. The relatives of the alcoholic will also need support and advice on how best they can help the patient to regain his good health.

NEOPLASTIC CONDITIONS

Benign tumours

These are rarely found in the liver, but may be an adenoma, fibroma or haemangioma. The tumours present as palpable nodules, usually do not give rise to symptoms and therefore are of no clinical significance. Treatment is not required.

Malignant tumours

Primary lesion (hepatoma)
Primary malignant tumours of the liver occur far less often than

secondary ones. The hepatoma is mainly associated with cirrhosis, and is a tumour of the hepatic cells. The cause is unknown but it is thought to be a toxic not a nutritional cause. The hepatoma may present as a solitary tumour or as a series of small ones, the right lobe of the liver being more often affected than the left. Metastases are likely to develop in other organs due to blood–borne or lymphatic spread, secondary lesions occurring in the lungs, brain, bones and the regional and mediastinal lymph nodes.

The patient may experience abdominal distension, pain in the right upper quadrant of the abdomen and gastrointestinal disturbances such as dyspepsia and anorexia. Jaundice may be present and there is often a slight rise in the temperature. Ascites occurs and the fluid may be bloodstained. Sometimes hypoglycaemia is present and may be due to the increased carbohydrate metabolism by the tumour. The tumour may invade the portal vein and give rise to portal hypertension, also the inferior vena cava may become obstructed. Primary malignant tumour of the liver is a rapidly progressive condition, and often death ensues within about four months of a diagnosis having been made.

Secondary lesions (metastases)
These occur about twenty times more frequently than hepatoma and develop from a primary lesion elsewhere in the gastrointestinal tract, the malignant cells being carried to the liver in the portal vein. Primary growths in other organs such as the lungs, breast and bronchus may metastasize to the liver in the systemic circulation and reach their destination in the hepatic artery. Men are more commonly affected than women. The patient may experience abdominal distension and epigastric pain; later jaundice and ascites may be present. Blood tests will show a rise in the alkaline phosphatase and transaminase levels. Secondary tumour in the liver will cause progressive deterioration in the patient's condition but this is usually not as rapid as for the primary lesion.

Treatment of malignant tumours
Much of the treatment for hepatic tumours is of necessity only

palliative due to the advanced stage of the primary lesion when the presence of metastases is confirmed, but if a diagnosis is made earlier then surgery may be undertaken with a moderate degree of success. With the aid of such investigations as hepatic arteriography, splenic venography and an inferior vena cavagram, together with a liver scan it should be possible to demonstrate the exact location of the tumour (or tumours) and thus help the surgeon to decide whether operation is feasible. The operation may be hepatic lobectomy or sub-total hepatectomy, for as much as ninety per cent of the liver may be removed as the remaining tissue shows great powers of regeneration which may be sufficient to reach a normal functional level. If surgery is contraindicated then the most usual treatment will be continuous liver perfusion into the hepatic artery using cytotoxic drugs; giving these systemically does not have the required effect. Finally, some success has been achieved with liver transplant, but there is still much to be learnt and accomplished in this respect, but it certainly gives encouragement that such treatment of neoplasms in the future will prove successful.

CHAPTER 6

The Biliary Tract

DEVELOPMENT AND ANATOMY OF THE GALL BLADDER

Position

During early fetal life the gall bladder is situated entirely within the liver, but later comes to lie in a fossa on the under surface of the right lobe of the liver, its position extending from the porta hepatis to the inferior border of the liver. The porta hepatis is the place of entry of the portal vein, hepatic artery and nerve plexus into the liver

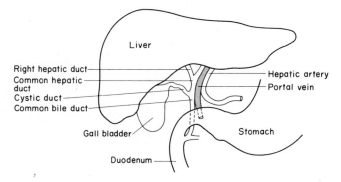

Fig. 31. *Gall bladder and related structures.*

128

and the exit of the two hepatic ducts and lymph vessels. The upper surface is attached to the liver by connective tissue, whereas the under surface and sides of the gall bladder are covered by peritoneum continued from the surface of the liver; thus the gall bladder is a retroperitoneal organ. Certain variations are found with regard to the position and relations of the gall bladder, and sometimes it is entirely covered by peritoneum and attached to the liver by a short mesentery.

Intrauterine development

At about the fourth week of embryonic life the foregut distal to the stomach and near its opening into the yolk sac gives rise to several diverticula; one of these, the hepatic diverticulum will eventually form the glandular tissue of the liver; two others will form the gall bladder and cystic duct and the pancreas. At this stage the pancreas is developing as two structures, a dorsal and ventral pancreas, the latter together with the common bile duct migrate around the duodenum from its right side to come to lie in the curve of the duodenum, and fusion of the two halves of the pancreas takes place.

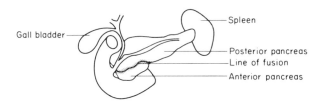

Fig. 32. *Fusion of two parts of the pancreas.*

The common bile duct thus passes downwards behind the first part of the duodenum and may be completely embedded in the pancreatic tissue, until at the second part of the duodenum it is joined by the pancreatic duct and together they form an ampulla (ampulla of Vater) which opens into the duodenum about 8–10 cm from the pylorus. This opening is guarded by a sphincter (sphincter of Oddi) which can act independently of the duodenal musculature.

The embryo undergoes flexion in the sagittal and transverse planes which results in some of the yolk sac being pinched up into the body of the embryo (Fig. 33), the surrounding mesoderm gives rise to various structures, one of these being the mesenteries which

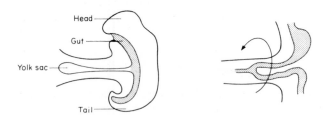

Fig. 33. *Early rotation of the gut; left-hand figure shows embryonic gut before rotation; right-hand, after rotation.*

suspend the gut in the coelomic cavity (Fig. 34). The gut distal to the stomach comes to be supported by the dorsal mesentery which attaches it to the dorsal abdominal wall. At this stage of development the gall bladder and biliary ducts are solid structures, canaliza-

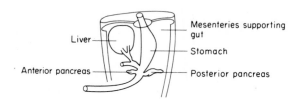

Fig. 34. *Gut suspended in coelomic cavity.*

tion occurs later by about the twelfth week of intrauterine life. Subsequently the ducts become hyperplastic and the lumen is obliterated, only to be recanalized by about the twentieth week of fetal life.

Blood supply

The three parts of the gut are vascularized by different arteries as the embryonic vascular system develops; the foregut, being that part of the gut which gives rise to all the structures of the alimentary tract as far as the entry of the common bile duct into the duodenum, receives its supply from the coeliac artery. Branches of this artery supply the gall bladder and ducts, the main one being the cystic artery which arises from the right hepatic artery. The cystic vein which is formed from vessels which accompany the branches of the cystic artery empties into the right branch of the portal vein.

Lymphatic supply

Situated alongside the bile ducts are lymphatic vessels, which together with those draining the gall bladder converge on the porta hepatis and empty into the hepatic nodes.

Nerve supply

The main nerve supply of the gall bladder is sympathetic, the fibres being derived from the coeliac plexus and passing in close association with the branches of the hepatic artery. Parasympathetic fibres from the hepatic branch of the vagus nerve also supply the gall bladder. From the hepatic plexus branches from the right phrenic nerve reach the gall bladder. This distribution is made apparent by referred pain to the right shoulder experienced by some with gall bladder conditions. The gall bladder empties by a mechanism thought to be under the control of a hormone (cholecystokinin), nervous stimulation not being entirely responsible for the contraction of the muscle wall.

PHYSIOLOGY OF THE GALL BLADDER

Concentration of bile

The gall bladder being 7–10 cm in length and about 3 cm in width is capable of holding only about 30–50 ml, hence one of its functions is to concentrate bile during its time of storage. This concentration of bile is achieved by the absorption of water and inorganic salts through its mucous lining, causing the bile to become darker in colour. This layer is thrown into rugae which increases the surface area as well as allowing for distension of the organ, and is continuous throughout the ducts leading both into the liver and down into the duodenum. By the absorption of bicarbonate, the pH of the bile leaving the gall bladder is lowered to about 7, compared with pH 8·2 of bile as it is received from the liver. The epithelial cells of the gall bladder lining secrete mucus, about 20 ml being produced each day, and this adds to the viscosity of the bile. If the biliary tract becomes obstructed distal to the cystic duct this process of concentration continues, the resulting bile taking on a tarry consistency which predisposes to the formation of gall stones.

Movements of the gall bladder

A rise in pressure in the gall bladder shortly after a meal is taken results in a proportion of the stored bile being discharged into the duodenum. After this initial flow bile is released intermittently, a small quantity at a time. Following the taking of a fatty meal the gall bladder decreases to one-fifth of its original size within half an hour. The fat content of the chyme is thought to stimulate the production of an enzyme, the active principle of which has been named cholecystokinin. This protein is related to secretin and is released into the blood stream from the duodenal mucosa. Stimulation of the gall bladder to contract and the sphincter of Oddi to relax is therefore mainly dependent on hormonal control. Some nervous stimulation of this mechanism is apparent when the rate of emptying is compared before and after complete vagotomy; following operation the gall bladder wall relaxes so that the volume of bile stored is increased and emptying occurs more slowly. If the hepatic branches of the vagus nerve are left intact then these changes are not apparent.

CONGENITAL CONDITIONS OF THE BILIARY APPARATUS

Congenital anomalies of the gall bladder occur in about ten per cent of persons, diagnosis usually being made following radiological examination. In many cases, an abnormality of the biliary apparatus gives rise to no symptoms and therefore, this is of importance only during surgery, whereas other anomalies are more serious and, despite attempts to reconstruct the gall bladder and its ducts, are not compatible with life.

Congenital anomalies of the gall bladder include:

Absence of the gall bladder

This is a rare condition, and is often associated with other abnormalities of the biliary tract. In about half the cases, it has been noted that gall stones are present in the common bile duct.

Double gall bladder

The diverticulum which gives rise to the gall bladder divides into

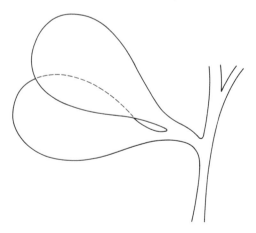

Fig. 35. *Double gall bladder.*

two, although the cystic duct remains single. One of the gall bladders is situated within the liver substance, and as they are likely to be diseased, removal of both is indicated.

Floating gall bladder

The gall bladder is attached to the liver by a mesentery which may

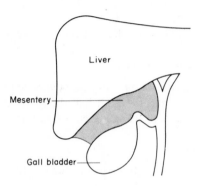

Fig. 36. *Floating gall bladder.*

be 2–3 cm in length. Because of this torsion may occur which leads to infarction in the blood vessels supplying the gall bladder.

Abnormalities of the cystic duct

These include absence of the cystic duct whereby the gall bladder opens directly into the common bile duct, or the duct may be excessive in length and opens into the common bile duct near the pancreas. Both of these conditions are of importance to the surgeon, the first because the common bile duct may be injured as the gall bladder is removed, and the second because if the cystic duct is not completely removed it can give rise to a return of symptoms.

Folded gall bladder

This abnormality results in kinking between the body and fundus of the gall bladder and is probably due to incomplete canalization of the cystic diverticulum in the embryo. It occurs in about 20% of normal healthy persons.

Accessory bile ducts

The gall bladder is connected to the liver by an extra duct which is only of importance following removal of the gall bladder where leakage of bile continues.

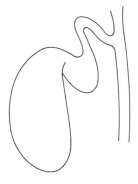

Fig. 37. *Folded gall bladder.*

Congenital atresia of the bile ducts

Various types of obstruction of the bile ducts may occur which include absence of a lumen or a narrowed lumen due to blockage of the duct by epithelial cell debris and bile filled cysts. The cause of these anomalies is probably due to a failure of canalization of the cystic diverticulum giving rise to various lengths of solid ducts. The liver enlarges and shows varying degrees of biliary cirrhosis. The baby may appear slightly jaundiced at birth, or jaundice develops within two to three days or sometimes not until the baby is several weeks old. The baby passes normal greenish-black meconium (formed about the twelfth to sixteenth week of intrauterine life) at first, but this is followed by pale clay coloured stools. The liver continues to enlarge, becomes hard on palpation, and death occurs as a result of hepatic failure or haemorrhage, the latter due to hypo-prothrombinaemia, or varices. The baby may thrive fairly well on a diet containing little fat, but without surgery death occurs at about six months. Some cases may be improved by surgery, and the differential diagnosis of the condition from other causes of neonatal jaundice (such as erythroblastosis fetalis, congenital spherocytosis) is preceded by liver function tests and liver biopsy (*see* page 104). If surgery is undertaken then the correction of dehydration, blood transfusion and the administration of vitamin K are necessary preoperatively. Prophylactic antibiotic therapy is usually given. Surgery may entail creating an opening between the gall bladder and jejunum (cholecystojejunostomy), but this is suitable only if the atresia is at the lower end of the common bile duct and the gall bladder and cystic duct are of normal appearance.

TRAUMA TO THE BILARY APPARATUS

Rupture of the gall bladder and biliary ducts

This is rare but may be acquired by a penetrating wound or crushing-type accident; occasionally operative techniques are responsible (*see* page 148). The ruptured gall bladder gives rise to features similar to that of perforation of the small intestine, with the addition of jaundice which becomes apparent within two to three hours of the accident. Treatment varies, and includes removal of the gall bladder, end to end anastomosis of the ducts together with drainage of bile from the peritoneal cavity.

Torsion of the gall bladder

This may occur where the congenital anomaly of a floating gall bladder exists. The patient experiences a sudden sharp pain, vomits and signs of shock are evident. The gall bladder may become gangrenous or rupture. The condition is relieved by removal of the gall bladder.

INFLAMMATORY CONDITIONS

Acute cholecystitis

The route by which organisms reach the gall bladder is uncertain but it is thought they travel in the blood, or in the lymphatics from the liver and intestines, in bile as it flows through the normal biliary channels, or by direct invasion from infected neighbouring organs. Acute cholecystitis rarely occurs as a primary infection of the gall bladder; in the majority of instances it is associated with obstruction to the neck of the gall bladder or cystic duct, which is most frequently due to gall stones (cholelithiasis), or sometimes oedema or obstruction by tumours. Mucosal damage which gives rise to oedema may result from reflux of pancreatic secretions containing destructive enzymes. The condition may also occur without obstruction being present, as is found in typhoid and paratyphoid fever. The organisms usually responsible for acute cholecystitis are streptococci (*Streptococcus faecalis, Streptococcus viridans*) and *Escherischia coli*, although in certain circumstances *Salmonella typhi* may be isolated.

The infected gall bladder appears very congested and haemorrhagic lesions may be present. Oedema of the wall causes the organ to be distended, and it is filled with turbid, and sometimes purulent bile (empyema of the gall bladder). Gangrene may result, leading to perforation and peritonitis, or the condition may pass into a chronic phase.

Clinical features

Acute cholecystitis is a condition which may occur at any age, but is most frequently seen in obese women of between forty and sixty years. It can occur in both sexes, the incidence being roughly equal if it occurs in old age.

Acute cholecystitis due to obstruction gives rise to a sudden onset of severe pain in the right hypochondrium. This is accompanied by nausea, vomiting and pyrexia of 38°C (100°F) or more, often with rigors. On examination of the abdomen, pain is most severe when a deep breath is taken, and a palpable mass is felt, consisting of the inflamed gall bladder. Jaundice may or may not be present, if it is then obstruction of the cystic duct is suggested. The patient may give a history of attacks of abdominal pain over recent weeks or months.

Diagnosis

It is important that acute cholecystitis should be differentiated from other causes of upper abdominal pain; these include acute appendicitis, duodenal ulcer, acute pyelonephritis and in some instances myocardial infarction. A plain abdominal X-ray has limited value but may show radio-opaque calculi, whereas a cholecystogram (*see* page 289) performed when the acute phase is passing may confirm the diagnosis.

Treatment

In the majority of cases the symptoms subside within a few days following conservative treatment, removal of the gall bladder (cholecystectomy) being carried out six to ten weeks later. At all times the nurse should be observing the patient for any change in the condition, particularly an increase in pain or rise in pulse rate, which might result in complications and therefore a need for immediate surgical treatment. If there is doubt as to the exact diagnosis then conservative treatment should not be undertaken and the gall bladder is removed at the outset. Some surgeons favour this as routine treatment for all cases of acute cholecystitis, provided surgery can be performed within forty-eight hours of the onset of symptoms.

Conservative treatment consists mainly of the following: relief of pain, relief of spasm, chemotherapy, rest to the gall bladder and dietetic treatment.

Relief of pain. This may be achieved by an injection of morphine sulphate 15–20 mg subcutaneously, or pethidine hydrochloride 100 mg intramuscularly. Although the former drug is known to cause contraction of the sphincter of Oddi, if it is given in a sufficiently large dose it is excellent as a means of relieving biliary colic. Some doctors do not favour its use, and would therefore prescribe pethidine. In any case due regard must be paid to the age of the patient in relation to the dose prescribed. The local application of heat by means of an electric pad, or suitably protected hot water bottle may be of comfort to the patient.

Relief of spasm. An anticholinergic drug such as propantheline bromide 30 mg intramuscularly may be used. This will have the effect of reducing the amount of gastric and pancreatic secretions, thus preventing the loss of important electrolytes by constant aspiration.

Chemotherapy. An antibiotic or chemotherapeutic agent is usually prescribed when pyrexia is present. Ampicillin 500 mg six hourly or tetracycline 500 mg six hourly may be given intravenously at first, changing to oral administration as soon as fluids by mouth are tolerated.

Rest to the gall bladder. In the initial phase this is achieved by allowing no food or fluids by mouth, and by passing an intragastric tube and aspirating the stomach contents at intervals. An intravenous infusion of dextrose saline with normal saline, is given during this time to maintain the electrolyte and fluid balance, the type of fluid and quantity given depending on the results of daily blood investigations. This treatment may be required for about three days after which as the symptoms subside the infusion can be discontinued, the intragastric tube removed, and the patient allowed to take small quantities of a fat free fluid at frequent intervals. Ambulation should now be encouraged.

Dietetic treatment

In the intervening weeks before surgery is undertaken, the patient will find that foods of a low fat content or that have not been cooked by frying, will prevent the return of symptoms. Some fat in the form of milk and butter should be included in the diet as this will encourage the gall bladder to empty, thus preventing stasis of bile which is thought to predispose to the formation of biliary calculi. Care may need to be exercised with regard to the carbohydrate content of the diet as many of these patients are overweight.

Chronic cholecystitis

This condition may have an insidious onset and progress slowly, or it may occasionally be the end result of acute cholecystitis. In about 90% of cases it is due to partial obstruction of the biliary passages by calculi. The gall bladder wall becomes thickened by fibrous tissue, the mucosal lining is scarred and atrophic with deep cystic spaces present in the wall. The bile often contains calculi. Sometimes an incomplete septum forms across the gall bladder dividing it into two chambers, one appears normal and the other has marked hypertrophy of the wall (cholecystitis glandularis proliferans). Diverticulosis of the gall bladder may also occur, black pigmented stones becoming impacted in the normal hollows of the gall bladder wall.

The majority of patients with these conditions present with biliary dyspepsia or occasionally an acute attack occurs. Diagnosis is by cholangiography (*see* page 290) and treatment usually involves removal of the gall bladder.

Cholelithiasis (gall stones)

These are present in about 10% of the adult population, but are rare before the age of forty years, occurring on average four times more frequently in females.

The factors responsible for the formation of calculi are metabolic factors, infection and stasis.

Metabolic factors

These calculi are due to changes in the composition of bile as excreted by the liver. Cholesterol is precipitated when it reaches a level of 13:1 in ratio to bile salts (normal ratio is 25:1). The bile salt level may fall as a result of dietary factors or infection in the gall bladder; this latter causes absorption of bile salts. The cholesterol stone is often large (1–5 cm in diameter), solitary, pale yellow in colour and may be translucent. On section the stone has a glistening appearance and the interior tends to radiate.

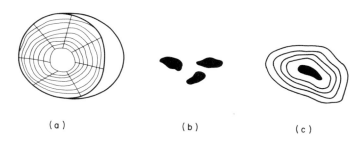

(a)   (b)   (c)

Fig. 38. *Stones, (a) metabolic stone (section shows radiating arrangement of pigments); (b) pigment stone (small, black); (c) mixed stone.*

Calcium bilirubinate gives rise to pigment stones which are jet black in colour, small, ovoid and often faceted. They are usually found in the common bile duct and are associated with increased haemolysis of red cells and the excretion by the liver of these breakdown products.

Mixed stones constitute about 80–90% of gall stones, and are composed of alternating layers of cholesterol and calcium bilirubinate, or cholesterol and calcium carbonate, together with a protein derived from the gall bladder. These calculi are always multiple, often faceted and vary in size and colour. Because they contain calcium they are usually radio-opaque.

Infection

Streptococci, coliform or typhoid organisms are frequently found in biliary calculi. On reaching the gall bladder the organism forms a focus to which mucosal cells become attached and later cholesterol and bile salts are added to complete the formation of the stone.

Stasis

Prevention of the normal flow of bile through the biliary tract will result in the increase in the size of stones which are forming. This situation may occur in pregnancy.

Sites of calculi

The majority of calculi are to be found in the gall bladder, but they may be present in other parts of the biliary tract, especially the common bile duct.

Effects of calculi

(1) Give rise to no symptoms.

(2) Cause biliary dyspepsia.

(3) Cause acute cholecystitis, or potentiate chronic cholecystitis.

(4) Obstruct the cystic duct, either completely or incompletely.

(5) Obstruct the common bile duct, either completely or incompletely.

(6) Pass into the small intestine and give rise to acute intestinal obstruction.

TUMOURS OF THE BILIARY TRACT

Benign tumours

These rare tumours are usually a papilloma or adenoma. The adenoma of the gall bladder may be associated with cholecystitis glandularis proliferans (see page 140). Benign tumours may give rise to obstructive jaundice.

Malignant tumours

Carcinoma of the gall bladder
This condition is uncommon, occurring in women more frequently than men, usually aged sixty to seventy years. Calculi and chronic cholecystitis predispose to this condition, the frequent irritation of the gall bladder mucosa probably potentiating the formation of a squamous cell carcinoma.

The patient may give a history of biliary dyspepsia over many years, associated with upper abdominal pain which has now become more severe and continuous. In many instances a large mass can be palpated in the area of the gall bladder. The common bile duct becomes completely obstructed by the tumour, either by compression or direct invasion; this results in obstructive jaundice. Other features include loss of weight, pyrexia and vomiting. Spread from the primary carcinoma may occur to the liver, lymphatic nodes in the porta hepatis and to the lungs.

Removal of the gall bladder in the early stages of the condition may prove successful.

Carcinoma of the extrahepatic biliary ducts
These tumours are rare, and occur even less frequently than those of the gall bladder. There is a gradual increase in jaundice, leading eventually to complete obstructive jaundice. Pain is common. The tumour is an adenocarcinoma, although calculi and inflammation do not appear to be a large factor in its formation.

The patient usually survives only a few months following diagnosis, as operative treatment is rarely possible.

SURGICAL TECHNIQUES

Cholecystectomy

Removal of the gall bladder is usually undertaken through a right paramedian incision. The cystic duct is ligated and divided close to its junction with the common bile duct and the gall bladder is dissected from its bed on the under surface of the liver, if possible leaving a flap of peritoneum to be sutured over the gall bladder bed. It is usual to drain the operation site by means of a 'stab' wound drainage tube inserted a little distance from the closure of the abdominal wall.

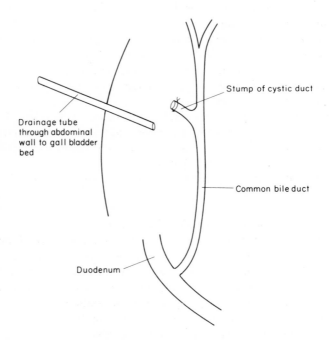

Stump of cystic duct

Drainage tube through abdominal wall to gall bladder bed

Common bile duct

Duodenum

Fig. 39. *Drainage of gall bladder bed following cholecystectomy.*

Cholecystostomy

This is an operation to remove stones from the gall bladder, and may be followed subsequently by cholecystectomy. Following the evacuation of the stones a drainage tube is passed into the gall bladder and then brought to the surface through a 'stab' incision.

The tubing is connected to a sterile polythene drainage bag. Provided there is no pyrexia and the stools are of normal colour the drainage tube is removed in 7–10 days time following cholangiography which will show the radio-opaque fluid passing unobstructed into the common bile duct and duodenum. The biliary fistula closes spontaneously.

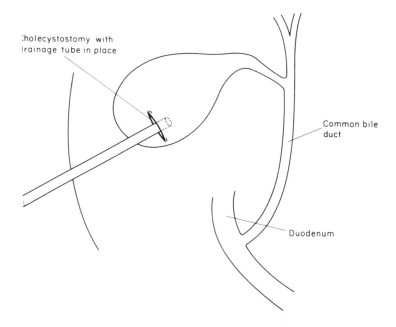

Fig. 40. *Gall bladder drainage.*

Choledochotomy

This procedure is carried out if stones are present in the common bile duct. The exploration of the bile duct can be approached by either of two routes, the supraduodenal, used when the stones can be manoeuvred into a position about half-way between the cystic duct

and the duodenum; and the transduodenal approach used when a
stone is impacted near the ampulla of Vater. If the stone is easily felt,
the common bile duct can be opened directly over it and the stone
removed (choledocholithotomy).

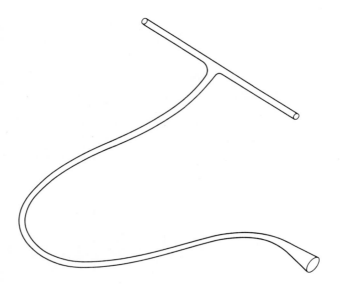

Fig. 41. *T-tube.*

It is usual to complete the operation of choledochotomy by
irrigating the common bile duct to remove grit, testing the patency
of the duct by an operative cholangiogram, and finally draining the
bile duct by means of a T-tube (Fig. 41). The tube is inserted into
the common bile duct, the stem of the T being brought out through a
'stab' incision and connected to a polythene drainage bag (choledo-

chostomy). This latter procedure is frequently carried out as a sequel to cholecystectomy.

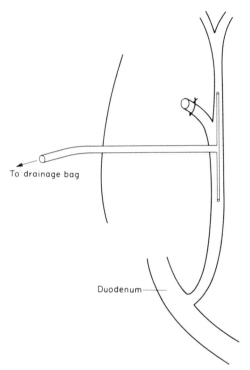

Fig. 42. *T-tube in position in common bile duct following choledochotomy and cholecystectomy.*

Choledochoduodenostomy

This operation entails the making of an incision in the wall of the common bile duct at its lower end, and suturing this to a similar incision made in a nearby part of the duodenum. The object of this procedure is to facilitate the passage of bile into the duodenum when the ampulla of Vater has become damaged by previous operative techniques, if there is doubt as to whether all stones have been removed, or if there is stricture at the lower end of the common bile duct and acute pancreatitis.

Biliary fistulae

These may be divided into external and internal fistulae.

External biliary fistulae

These fistulae usually follow operation on the biliary tract. The discharge will be mucus if the gall bladder or cystic duct is occluded, and bile if a stone blocks the common bile duct following cholecystectomy. In either case the cause must be found (by means of a cholangiogram), and either the gall bladder removed or the patency of the common bile duct restored.

Internal biliary fistulae

Internal biliary fistulae are due to stones ulcerating through the wall of the gall bladder or common bile duct into an adjacent organ such as the duodenum, colon or stomach. The fistula may close spontaneously, but the stone may cause obstruction. Surgery will be required.

Complications of gall bladder surgery

Stricture

This may occur in either the common hepatic duct or common bile duct following an attempt to control bleeding from the cystic artery. The instrument used clamps not only the bleeding point but also the bile duct, resulting in permanent damage. Stricture of the common bile duct may occur during partial gastrectomy.

Laceration

The common bile duct may be lacerated whilst it is being explored for gall stones.

The majority of these complications are preventable by employing good operative techniques. The effects may not be noted for several days post-operatively until the patient continues to become more jaundiced, the drainage of bile more profuse or peritonitis results.

SPECIFIC NURSING CARE

Pre-operative care

The specific investigations carried out before operation will include blood tests and radiology.

Blood tests

Blood group, haemoglobin and electrolyte levels will be noted. In cases of acute pancreatitis the serum amylase level will be estimated; this may be raised to 800 units/100 ml blood (normal 80–150 units/100 ml blood). The prothrombin time may be increased to 30 or more seconds (normal 12–15 seconds) indicating a lack of vitamin K in the liver for its manufacture, and therefore an increased tendency to bleeding. The serum bilirubin level may be estimated by the Van den Bergh test, and may be 0–85 μmol/l (0–5 mg%) (normal 0·2–0·8 mg%).

Radiological investigations

These may include plain abdominal and chest films, cholecystogram (*see* page 289) or intravenous cholangiogram (*see* page 290). Following the latter, the nurse should observe the patient for side effects such as restlessness, nausea, vomiting and a sensation of upper abdominal pressure.

The preparation of the patient for surgery should include the administration of vitamin K in the form of phytomenadione (Konakion) 10 mg daily for 5 days to patients undergoing surgery for obstructive jaundice, breathing exercises, an abdominal shave, and the passage of an intragastric tube (if requested by the surgeon).

Post-operative care

The importance of the care of the unconscious patient cannot be over emphasized. The nurse should constantly note the patient's colour, and respiratory and pulse rate in particular.

Some patients may not be allowed fluids by mouth during the first 24–36 hours: an intravenous infusion of 5% dextrose, or dextrose saline and normal saline may be given during this time. These patients will probably have had an intragastric tube passed, which will require aspirating at half to one hourly intervals, or more often if nausea is experienced. As the amount of aspirate becomes less the interval between aspirating can be increased until the tube is removed on the second or third post-operative day. Where intravenous fluids and gastric aspirations are not indicated, once consciousness is regained, the patient will be allowed fluids by mouth, gradually increasing the quantity given at any one time until an adequate amount of fluid and a light diet is taken by about the third post-operative day. Following cholecystectomy the diet should be low in fat content at first, but the patient should be encouraged to eat a normal diet as soon as possible.

Management of drainage tubes

The drainage tube to the gall bladder may be shortened on the day following operation, and then daily until it is removed on the third to fifth post-operative day. The dressing should be renewed as necessary.

The drainage from the T-tube should be measured and recorded. Variations exist as to the position of the drainage bag in relation to the patient. Some surgeons have the bag below the level of the patient for a few days, then raised to a position higher than the gall bladder site for several days allowing drainage to continue throughout this time; whilst others have the drainage interrupted by applying a clip to the tubing each day for increasing intervals from about the fifth day onwards, until finally the tube is clipped off for twenty-four hours. Whichever method is used and provided the patient's stools are of normal colour, the urine free from bile and biliary drainage decreasing, a cholangiogram is usually performed through the T-tube on about the tenth post-operative day, and if this indicates a normal passage of bile into the duodenum the tube is removed. Before removal of the tube the patient may require an analgesic such as intramuscular pethidine hydrochloride 50–100 mg, the suture securing the tube will be cut, and the tube removed by steady traction. There is likely to be some escape of bile along the fistula during the next few days; dressings should be renewed as necessary until the fistula closes. Continuous contact of bile with the skin will cause excoriation, and if the flow is not decreasing some protective application such as aluminium compound paste will be necessary.

Patients undergoing surgery on the biliary tract usually experience a considerable amount of pain post-operatively. This may prevent adequate chest movement and coughing which coupled with the tendency to obesity may make the patient reluctant to move and get up out of bed. These activities should be encouraged, and adequate analgesia given to facilitate them with the minimum of discomfort.

CHAPTER 7

The Pancreas

The pancreas is a mixed gland producing both an exocrine and endocrine secretion. It is leaf-shaped 10–15 cm in length, consisting of a head, body and tail, and yellow in colour with a slight reddish hue. The head of the pancreas nestles snugly in the curve of the duodenum, the gland extending transversely across the abdomen to the spleen at the level of the first to second lumbar vertebra. The pancreas lies deep in the epigastric and left hypochondriac areas of the abdomen, behind the peritoneum forming the lesser omental sac.

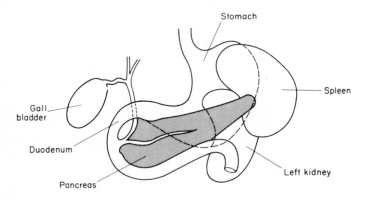

Fig. 43. *Pancreas and related structures.*

The common bile duct passes either through a groove formed by the gland and the adjacent curve of the duodenum, or through the actual substance of the gland. Anteriorly the pyloric antrum of the stomach and the transverse colon are found over the head of the pancreas, whilst posteriorly the inferior vena cava, left renal vein and aorta are located. The body of the pancreas tapers into a short tail which fits into the hilum of the spleen and is in contact with the left kidney on its posterior surface.

Embryology and physiology

Diverticula grow out from the wall of that part of the foregut which later will become the duodenum, in both a dorsal and ventral direction. From each diverticulum chains of constantly dividing cells form cellular cords; the tips of these cords remain solid, later separating from the main cord and differentiating to form the endocrine tissue. The remainder of the cord cannalizes and will eventually form the exocrine pancreatic cells. The original diverticula and their main branches will form the duct system of the pancreas, surrounded by connective tissue, capillary and lymphatic vessels. As development proceeds the stomach and duodenum rotate which causes the ventral pancreas to pass behind the duodenum and to come to lie alongside and beneath the larger dorsal diverti-

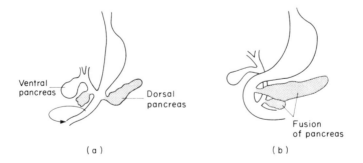

Ventral pancreas

Dorsal pancreas

Fusion of pancreas

(a)   (b)

Fig. 44. *Development of pancreas: (a) before rotation of gut; (b) after rotation of gut.*

F

culum of the pancreas. Fusion of the two diverticula takes place and the resulting pancreas is situated within the curve of the duodenum.

The duct systems of the two diverticula intercommunicate, the ventral portion forming the head of the pancreas, and the dorsal part the body and tail, the greater part of the ducts of this latter diverticulum forming the main pancreatic duct. As the stomach rotates it causes the peritoneal layer on the posterior aspects of the pancreatic diverticula to come into contact with parietal peritoneum over the posterior abdominal wall. As the ventral and dorsal pancreas fuses, it becomes flattened in shape and adherent to the posterior abdominal wall, causing the two peritoneal layers now in contact to fuse and later become obliterated. Thus the pancreas now occupies a retroperitoneal position, with peritoneum attached along its anterior surface and superior edge of the tail of the pancreas (this peritoneum forms the posterior layer of the lesser omental sac). The tail of the pancreas is now located and fixed in the lienorenal ligament which attaches the spleen to the posterior abdominal wall. The main pancreatic duct (of Wirsung) passes centrally through the organ draining the tail and body as it passes towards the papilla of Vater where it enters the duodenum, either through a separate orifice or sharing an opening with the common bile duct. The sphincter of Oddi closes both ducts preventing reflux of intestinal contents. Several accessory ducts (including the duct of Santorini) may be present which drain parts of the head of the pancreas and enter separately into the duodenum; these are subject to much anatomical variation as regards number and location.

The blood supply of the pancreas is derived mainly from the splenic artery which passes along and behind the upper border of the organ sending branches into the body and tail. The gastroduodenal artery which originates from the common hepatic artery passes downwards over the front of the head of the pancreas, whereas the many branches of the superior mesenteric artery anastomose to form a network surrounding the head of the pancreas and part of the duodenum. Venous drainage from the pancreas is by the superior and inferior mesenteric veins, the latter entering the splenic vein and the two then joining to form the portal vein which passes to the liver. The pancreas is supplied by branches of the vagus nerve, but its function is mainly controlled by hormonal factors.

Microscopically the pancreas is found to partly resemble the structure of a salivary gland, being made up of long tubular alveoli, the cells surrounding a narrow lumen when the alveolus is resting, but during activity the lumen becoming distended with secretion. The alveolar cells are packed with zymogen granules (the precursors of the pancreatic enzymes) in the inactive phase, the cells becoming empty of granules after release of secretion. Scattered

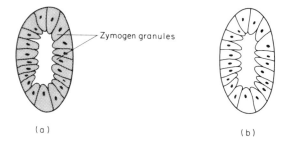

Zymogen granules

(a)   (b)

Fig. 45. *Pancreatic cells before and after hormonal stimulation; (a) resting pancreatic cells; (b) pancreatic cells after release of zymogen cells.*

amongst the alveolar tissue are found groups of epithelial cells without a duct which form the islets of Langerhans. These cells are mainly of two types, the more numerous beta cells which contain granules which are the precursors of insulin, and the less numerous alpha cells which possess the precursor of glucagon. The islets vary in size and are more numerous in the tail of the pancreas, the organ containing about a million of these areas of specialized tissue.

The pancreas contributes about 800 ml of juice daily to aid digestion in the small intestine, secretion being stimulated by the release of secretin, produced by the wall of the duodenum in response to the presence of acid chyme from the stomach. This hormone travels in the blood to stimulate the release of pancreatic juice and empty the alveoli of zymogen granules. Pancreatic secretion is alkaline in reaction with a pH 8·4 and contains the enzymes trypsinogen, chymotrypsinogen and peptidases which exert an action on protein, amylase and maltase which act on carbohydrate; as well as lipase and nuclease. The release of the hormone insulin from the islet cells is controlled by the circulating blood sugar level, the action of insulin being mainly to facilitate the entry of glucose into the cells and stimulate the conversion of excess glucose into glycogen for storage in the liver. Inability of the pancreas to produce sufficient insulin to maintain this balance leads to the condition of diabetes mellitus. Conversely, when the blood sugar level falls, glucagon is released from the pancreas to initiate the mobilization of glycogen in the liver to make it available for the body's needs.

CONGENITAL ANOMALIES

Gross anatomical malformations are rare but sometimes ectopic pancreatic tissue is found situated in the wall of the stomach or small intestine. The amount of tissue is small and usually does not give rise to symptoms, but just occasionally may be involved in intestinal obstruction. Anomalies of the pancreatic ducts may occur: the main duct may drain into the common bile duct or enter the duodenum above the ampulla of Vater. Other rare abnormalities are agenesis of the pancreas, failure of fusion of the dorsal and ventral portions of the pancreas to form one organ: the ventral portion may encircle the duodenum causing obstruction.

Congenital cystic disease of the pancreas

This condition (fibrocystic disease or mucoviscidosis) is one of the manifestations of a congenital abnormality of mucus secretion which can affect all mucus-secreting glands in the body. It has a high familial tendency and is one of three clinical types:

Meconium ileus
This is a condition of the newborn in which the meconium is pale

and viscid due to lack of pancreatic secretions, the ileum is dilated and intestinal obstruction occurs. Surgery to relieve the obstruction is not always successful.

Infantile type

This condition is usually apparent within a few weeks or months of birth, the infant fails to thrive and often suffers from dyspnoea and a cough. The bronchi become dilated and blocked by secretions, which lead to fibrosis and collapse of pulmonary tissue. At this stage death may occur from staphylococcal pneumonia or right sided heart failure. Steatorrhoea is usually present, the child frequently passing large greasy and offensive stools. The child is invariably hungry but remains extremely wasted in appearance.

Childhood type

The childhood type resembles coeliac disease in some respects. The child fails to thrive, the stools contain excess fat and lack pancreatic secretions when tested. Respiratory complications are a likely occurrence. In all types of fibrocystic disease there is an increase in the sodium chloride content of sweat, tears and saliva, a factor which can be tested for as an aid to diagnosis. Cirrhosis of the liver and portal hypertension may be present. With treatment the child may survive without gross pulmonary or hepatic damage, in which case the prognosis is improved.

Treatment consists of giving casein hydrolysate and pancreatin to replace the deficiency, together with additional vitamins and sodium chloride. Broad spectrum antibiotics will need to be used both as therapy and prophylaxis for respiratory infections.

TRAUMA

Injury to the pancreas is uncommon, but may occur along with damage to other abdominal organs following a road traffic accident, and will then be found during laparotomy. If the tail of the pancreas is nearly severed it is usually removed, whereas laceration of the head of the pancreas can be repaired by suturing. A fistula may result as a complication of this type of pancreatic injury.

Pancreatic fistula

This situation may follow trauma to the gland or occur as a complication following splenectomy. The management becomes both a surgical and nursing problem as any release of pancreatic enzymes onto the skin will quickly cause excoriation, and as much as two litres of fluid over a twenty-four hour period may be lost in this way. The fluid loss and electrolyte balance will need to be corrected, either by the oral or intravenous route, and then drainage from deep in the wound may be carried out through a tube attached to a suction pump. The pancreatic fluid can then be collected into a suitable container, the skin surrounding the drainage tube being cleaned frequently and protected by the application of a barrier cream such as aluminium paste or Stomaseal. Spontaneous closure of the fistula may occur, but this may not take place for weeks or months, and it is not surprising that the patient suffers periods of depression, particularly as the skin seems to be permanently wet and the dressings constantly to need changing. Continuous care and attention will be required by the patient, and the nurse must encourage both physical and mental activity to prevent periods of boredom. If the fistula fails to close, then it should be dissected down to its source and drained into the stomach or a loop of jejunum.

INFLAMMATORY CONDITIONS

Inflammation of the pancreas may be either acute or chronic, the former being a serious disorder which still carries a high mortality rate.

Acute pancreatitis

Acute pancreatitis may occur concurrently with other biliary tract disorders or following operation for them, or it may present as a complication of mumps, typhoid fever, malignant hypertension and alcoholism. Auto-digestion is the main feature of this condition, release of pancreatic enzymes allows the activation of trypsinogen. How this is brought about is uncertain but it may be due to obstruction of the pancreatic duct, infection, or reflux of bile and duodenal juice. The effect on the pancreas is that it becomes enlarged and firm with areas of haemorrhage and fat necrosis. Diagnostic tests will reveal a leucocytosis, and raised serum and urinary amylase levels often to over 1000 Somogyi units per 100 ml compared with the normal 80–150 units in the blood, and over 500 units (normal below 50) in the urine. The serum bilirubin level may be raised, and the serum calcium level falls, often to a dangerously low level. Acute pancreatitis may affect either male or female, thin or obese, but the patient is usually between fifty and sixty years and experiences the acute attack following the taking of alcohol or a large meal. Epigastric pain is severe and radiates through to the back, vomiting occurs and there is abdominal tenderness and rigidity. The patient may collapse and become cyanosed, with a lowered blood pressure. The features of this condition may be confused with perforation of a peptic ulcer, myocardial infarction or intestinal obstruction. It is therefore important that a correct differential diagnosis is made, assisted by blood tests and an electro-cardiograph.

Treatment and nursing care

Acute pancreatitis is treated conservatively as operation would only increase the mortality. Rest is essential, both for the patient and the pancreas. Aspiration of gastric juice by means of a nasogastric tube will help to relieve the feelings of nausea and reduce hormonal stimulation of the pancreas. No fluids are given by mouth, and hydration is maintained by the intravenous route. Propantheline may be given to reduce the activity of the vagus nerve. Relief of pain by the use of pethidine hydrochloride 100 mg intramuscularly should be given at the outset and repeated. Some surgeons prefer morphine not to be used as it increases the spasm of the sphincter of Oddi. Plasma may be given, along with calcium gluconate in an endeavour to restore the fluid and electrolyte balance. A broad spectrum antibiotic is usually prescribed. When the patient's condition improves fluids may be given by mouth, progressing to a light diet of small quantities of plain foods. Gastric aspiration and the intravenous regimen may then be discontinued. Now that the patient feels better, mobilization may be encouraged and the patient should attend to his personal care. Investigations of the biliary tract should be undertaken, but tests should be delayed for a few weeks to allow a period of convalescence. Surgery may be indicated when the result of the tests are known; this should be carried out so as to prevent a recurrence of pancreatitis.

Chronic pancreatitis

This occasionally follows an acute attack, or may result from a vascular disorder such as arteriosclerosis of the abdominal arteries or obstruction of the duct by calculi or stricture formation. Chronic pancreatitis is usually a slowly progressive disease of destruction of pancreatic tissue and its replacement by fibrosis. The main features of this chronic condition are pain, obstructive jaundice and diabetes mellitus due to inadequate endocrine secretion. Pain may not be continuous but occur in episodes with periods of remission. Treatment consists of giving a high protein, high calorie diet with additional vitamins. No alcohol should be taken. Treatment of diabetes and correction of anaemia, together with relief of pain by giving suitable analgesics, may cause the attacks to become less severe and more infrequent.

Cysts and calculi of the pancreas

True cysts of the pancreas are mainly congenital anomalies in development of the ducts, where variable sized cysts of fibrous tissue filled with a clear mucoid fluid occur, often forming part of polycystic disease and thus being associated with similar cysts in the liver and kidneys. Obstruction to the ducts and chronic pancreatitis may give rise to small thin walled retention cysts. Malignant tumours of the pancreas may originate from cystadenoma.

False cysts of the pancreas (pseudopancreatic cysts) are mainly large solitary collections of serous fluid, either within the pancreatic tissue or adjacent to it. Their cause is often unknown, but they may be present following acute pancreatitis or trauma. Fibrocystic disease is not a true cystic condition of the pancreas.

Pancreatic calculi occur in the older age group, the stones consisting of calcium carbonate and phosphate. They may not give rise to symptoms or may cause obstruction in a duct or chronic pancreatitis.

NEOPLASTIC CONDITIONS

Benign tumours

Benign tumours of the pancreas are rare, mainly they comprise the fibroma, lipoma and haemangioma, together with adenoma and cystadenoma. Islet cell tumours are also not common, but are important because of the hormonal effects which they cause. These are small firm nodules found mainly in the tail of the pancreas occurring more often in men aged between thirty and fifty years. The cells resemble those of the islets of Langerhans, being predominantly alpha and beta cells, some 60% of which are endocrinologically active. Tumours affecting the beta cells will be insulin secreting and give rise to symptoms of hypoglycaemia. Tumours of the alpha cells appear to secrete gastrin and not glucagon as might be expected, and this gives rise to the Zollinger–Ellison syndrome, in which peptic ulceration occurs in the duodenum and jejunum in the presence of a very high gastric acid secretion (*see* Chapter 4). Treatment is by surgical removal of the tumour.

Malignant tumours

Carcinoma of the pancreas is a moderately common tumour, occurring twice as frequently in men as in women of around sixty years of age. The majority, (70%), of neoplasms are situated in the head of the pancreas, although they may be found in the body and tail. Often the tumours are small, hard and white in appearance, giving rise to extensive metastases which are to be found in adjacent organs such as the duodenum and common bile duct, liver, lungs and peritoneum when ascites occurs, together with extensive lymphatic spread. Malignant tumours are of two types, the adenocarcinoma and the less common spheroidal cell tumour. The effects of carcinoma of the head of the pancreas are progressive obstructive jaundice leading to cirrhosis, obstruction and thrombosis in the portal vein and diabetes mellitus.

Symptoms in this condition vary. The patient may present with painless jaundice, or pain may occur prior to the onset of jaundice. The pain is felt in the epigastric region and radiates to the back and may be colicky in type and mimic gall stone pain. The patient complains of weakness, continuing loss of weight, anorexia and pruritus due to the jaundice. On examination, the liver is found to be palpable and enlarged. Diagnosis is assisted by examination of the stools, where occult blood is found to be present and the stercobilinogen content is reduced. Pancreatic biopsy may be carried out. Pancreatic scanning with the aid of radioactive isotopes may also be used to show a tumour.[75] Se-methionine is given intravenously and is well concentrated in the pancreas within an hour of injection. This isotope is also taken up by the liver, and so a separate liver scan

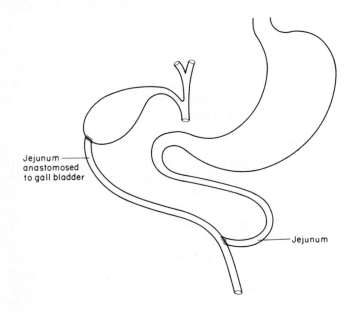

Jejunum anastomosed to gall bladder

Jejunum

Fig. 46. *Cholecystojejunostomy.*

using technetium (this is not taken up by the pancreas) will need to be done to clarify the situation. Diagnosis may not be confirmed until an exploratory laparotomy is undertaken, the results of this may prove the carcinoma to be inoperable, when a palliative procedure of anastomosing the gall bladder to the jejunum (cholecystojejunostomy) may be done in order that the flow of bile by-passes the pancreas. Some inoperable carcinomas show a reasonable response to the use of cytotoxic drugs. It is important that regular blood tests are made. If the situation appears to be operable then pancreatoduodenectomy may be performed. In this procedure the head of the pancreas is removed and the remaining pancreatic tissue anastomosed to the jejunum and the duodenum is removed. Blood transfusion will be necessary and also injection of vitamin K during the immediate post-operative days. Antibiotics should be given prophylactically. Total pancreatectomy is occasionally the operation of choice, this will necessitate the replacement of enzymes by giving pancreatin 10–12 g daily, also the insulin requirements will need to be assessed and replaced.

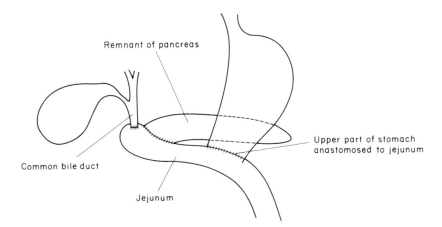

Fig. 47. *Pancreatoduodenectomy*.

Nursing care

The patient should be nursed in the sitting position as this tends to reduce the amount of pain experienced, especially in the back. Whichever operation has been performed a nasogastric tube will need to be passed and the gastric juices aspirated during the immediate post-operative period. Intravenous fluids should prevent dehydration and blood may need to be transfused to correct anaemia. As the patient is thin and weak, gentle mobilization should be encouraged, and help given with personal toilet care. A soothing local application or the use of antihistamines may help control the pruritus. Nausea may be a problem, but antiemetics such as metoclopramide 10 mg (Maxolon) may be effective; this is particularly so if the patient is having a course of cytotoxic drugs. Pain will need to be controlled by giving pethidine hydrochloride or pentazocine (Fortral) at first, and then less strong analgesics if they are found to be suitable. Constipation should be avoided, and suppositories may be necessary. The diet should be high protein and high calorie and may need to be given as smaller and more frequent meals. The prognosis for this condition is poor but some patients improve temporarily after surgery and the nurse should aim to help the patient improve to a state where he can be discharged from hospital even if only for a limited period.

CHAPTER 8

The Small Intestine

Development of the intestine

In an earlier chapter the development of the stomach was considered, and this was shown to have formed from the forepart of the embryonic gut; this same area gives rise to the proximal part of the duodenum, whereas the remainder of the small intestine and the large intestine, as far as the right two-thirds of the transverse colon, originate from the midgut. During the early development of the embryo the loop of midgut elongates rapidly, and together with the growing kidneys and enlarging liver almost fills the abdominal cavity; this results in the midgut together with its dorsal mesentery herniating into the umbilical cord. Whilst there the gut undergoes further development finally returning to the abdomen at about the twelfth week of fetal life. The growth of the midgut is not uniform along its length, the proximal part elongating faster than the distal and undergoing rotation, and when this re-enters the abdomen it occupies a position to the right of the future descending colon.

The distal part of the midgut re-enters the abdomen after the proximal part and this will give rise to the caecum and appendix, passing first to the right upper quadrant and occupying a position just underneath the liver, thus carrying the transverse colon across the abdomen to a position in front of the retroperitoneal duodenum. The duodenum was taken to the right side of the abdomen by the rotation of the foregut during the formation of the stomach, the

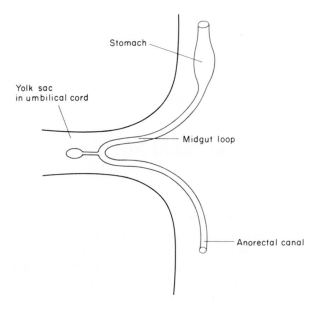

Fig. 48. *Loop of midgut in umbilical cord.*

former fused with the dorsal parietal peritoneum, lost its mesentery and became a retroperitoneal organ. Slowly the caecum grows, and as it does so, descends into the right iliac fossa taking the appendix with it.

The remainder of the colon, the rectum and upper part of the anal canal develop from the hindgut. The lower part of the anal canal forms from anal swellings which encircle the canal, their epithelial coverings becoming continuous with the endothelial lining of the hindgut at the site of rupture of the embryonic cloacal membrane. The upper and lower parts of the anal canal therefore have different types of epithelia (columnar cells line the upper part and squamous cells the lower) and different nerve innervation, vascular and lymphatic supply. During the early stages of development rapid proliferation of the gut wall causes the lumen of the gut to become

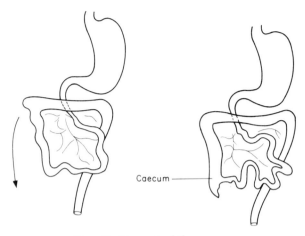

Fig. 49. *Descent of the caecum.*

obliterated, but later recanalization occurs which usually starts to take place at about the seventh or eighth week of fetal life. Epithelial cells line the lumen of the gut and extend along tubular ingrowths to the surrounding tissue, giving rise to cells which are secretory by

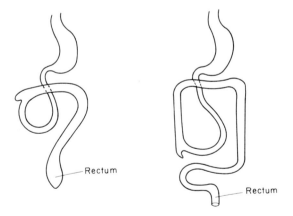

Fig. 50. *Development of the rectum.*

function and also form a lining of the ducts of the intestinal glands. The majority of the digestive enzymes are present by the twentieth week of fetal life and are to be found in full quantity by birth. Lack of any of these enzymes makes the baby intolerant of various sugars and leads to diarrhoea and failure to thrive.

In view of the complex manoeuvres which ultimately result in the formation of the gut it is no wonder that anomalies in development occasionally occur. Such outcomes may include:

(1) Mal- or non-rotation of the gut leading to abnormal positions of the viscera and mesenteries.

(2) The herniation of the midgut into the umbilical cord may persist (exomphalos) or coils of intestine may remain partly in the base of the umbilical cord (Meckel's diverticulum).

(3) Recanalization of the gut may be incomplete giving rise to atresia or stenosis at any level.

(4) Imperforate anus may result from failure of the anal membrane to break down.

(5) The urorectal septum may fail to grow, therefore fistulae between the rectum and bladder, urethra and vagina may result. Some urogenital organs also develop from the hindgut and become separated from it by the urorectal septum, the distal end of which forms the perineal body.

(6) Defective fixation of the duodenum and parts of the colon may result.

(7) The caecum may remain in position under the liver, and malposition of the peritoneum which normally anchors it in the right iliac fossa might allow volvulus of the whole of the small intestine to occur.

(8) The position of these abdominal organs may be reversed.

The diagnosis, treatment and related nursing care concerning some of these anomalies will be considered in the appropriate part of the text in this chapter and the next.

Movements of the small intestine

Movements of the small intestine are mainly of two kinds, segmentation and peristalsis.

Segmentation is the sudden and simultaneous contraction of the wall of the gut occurring at intervals which has the effect of dividing a length of gut into roughly equal segments. A few seconds later contraction occurs in the middle of each of these dilated areas and the previously contracted muscle relaxes, and thus a new set of segments are formed. The effect of this type of movement on the contents of the intestine is to assist thorough mixing of the chyme with the digestive juices and also to bring it into closer contact with the absorptive lining of the intestinal wall; it does not play any part in the movement of chyme through the gut towards the large intestine. Segmentation may occur as frequently as at five to ten second intervals in the duodenum immediately after the arrival of a meal there. A gradient of activity in the intestine is noted as segmentation occurs more slowly in the jejunum and even slower still in the ileum.

Peristalsis is a movement of the intestine which occurs in waves and results in the propulsion of foodstuffs along the gut. It is achieved by the contraction of circular muscle fibres (the inner layer of smooth muscle fibres in the wall of the gut) behind a mass of intestinal contents, this movement being preceded by relaxation of the muscular wall of the part of the gut into which the contents will be pushed. The gut is capable of peristaltic moves in one direction only, and the propulsive waves may occur up to twelve times per minute, commencing in the duodenum within minutes of starting to take a meal. The circular muscle layer forms the ileocolic sphincter at the entry to the caecum from the ileum; here food is held up after its passage through the small intestine which may have taken three to four hours. A portion of it at a time is allowed through when the sphincter opens momentarily before closing abruptly (this prevents backflow of the contents), and it may be some eight or nine hours following the meal before all food residue has passed into the large intestine. Although this part of the gut is innervated by the vagus nerve, the action of this sphincter is not affected by alterations in vagal stimulation. Meals of differing food constituents will vary in the time taken to pass through the small intestine. The motility of various parts of the intestine can be measured by picking up the signal emitted from a pressure sensitive transducer contained in a small capsule which is swallowed.

Intestinal mucosa

The average length of the small intestine is about 5 m (16 ft), which is reduced to just over 2 m (about 6 ft) by the tone in the muscles along the wall. The surface is then considerably increased by the presence of some five million villi making an area of ten square metres. The 'brush border' of the columnar epithelial cells which forms the outer layer of the villi further increases this area about thirty times. The jejunal villi are larger than those in the other parts of the small intestine. Muscle fibres from the muscularis mucosa enter the base of each villus and attach to the lacteal. Contraction of these fibres assists in the movements of the villi, a feature which is constantly happening during the process of digestion, and also helps the onward movement of the lymph. The mesenteric veins convey blood from the small intestine to the portal vein, and here just over one litre of blood flows through per minute, being increased by one-third during the digestion of a meal.

Digestion and absorption of nutrients

Although digestion normally starts in the mouth and is continued in the stomach the small intestine has the ability to cope with all foodstuffs if the former areas are by-passed. Digestion is largely carried out by the enzymes contained in pancreatic juice in conjunction with bile; the enzymes present in succus entericus secreted from Brunner's glands found only in the first part of the duodenum play a relatively small role. Carbohydrates are eventually broken down to their final products of simple monosaccharides, and as glucose, galactose and fructose are absorbed into the capillaries of the villi. Proteins in the chyme are broken down to polypeptides, and then to amino acids for absorption. The digestion and absorption of fats is more complex. Pancreatic lipase converts fats to fatty acids and glycerides, to be acted on by bile salts. This has the effect of dividing them into particle size, the small molecules (those less than 0.5μ in diameter) or short-chain fatty acids can be absorbed through the villus wall into the capillary and enter the blood stream through the portal circulation. The larger particles (greater than 0.5μ in diameter) or long-chain fatty acids enter the lacteal and are conveyed to the systemic circulation in the chyle. Fat probably enters the cells of the villi by pinocytosis (the engulfing of small particles by individual cells) through the 'brush border'. Many factors affect the absorption of fat including the degree of emulsification which has taken place. Usually about 95% of fat taken in in the diet is absorbed, and any defects can be measured by estimating the amount of fat present in the faeces during a given period of time following a known quantity of dietary fat having been taken. Where large quantities of fat fail to be absorbed the stools usually appear pale and bulky, the condition being known as steatorrhoea. Cholesterol is emulsified by bile salts and absorbed slowly into the lymphatics; related plant sterols are not absorbed. The presence of bile salts is necessary for the absorption of vitamins A, D, E and K by the small intestine. In the ileum vitamin B_{12} is absorbed with the aid of the intrinsic factor supplied by the stomach, to a maximum daily total of about 2 microgrammes. This is sufficient for the normal health of the individual.

Faulty mechanisms in the absorption of nutrients by the small intestine are collectively called the 'malabsorption syndrome'. The implications of this condition are discussed on page 174.

CONGENITAL ANOMALIES

Duodenal atresia

Atresia found in the small intestine occurs with highest incidence in the duodenum, then the ileum, jejunum and colon in descending order of frequency. In the duodenum the block in the lumen is usually just distal to the ampulla of Vater. This abnormality occurs in about 1 in 10 000 births, 50% of which are premature, and of these half have other congenital malformations affecting either the gut, kidneys, heart or skeletal structures. Thirty per cent of cases are also associated with Down's syndrome (mongolism). In the majority of instances there is a history of hydramnios occurring in pregnancy.

Typically, the baby appears healthy at first, meconium is usually passed within a few hours of birth and feeding is commenced. Vomiting then occurs after twenty-four or thirty-six hours, becoming persistent and containing bile in many instances. Unless a diagnosis is made and treatment instituted promptly the baby will quickly become dehydrated with an associated electrolyte imbalance. Diagnosis should be made by taking a plain X-ray film of the abdomen, and this will show the stomach and proximal part of the duodenum to be distended with air, a quite reverse situation to that noted in the remainder of the gut. It is both dangerous and unnecessary to do a barium X-ray on this baby. Prior to operation the baby should have a nasogastric tube passed and left in position (size 10 FG/4EG) and the stomach aspirated. A specimen of blood should be taken for investigation of electrolytes and blood group. An intravenous infusion should be set up preferably into a scalp vein, and blood for transfusion should be made available. Under general anaesthesia a laparotomy is performed and as much of the gut examined as possible as the duodenum may not be the only area affected. Depending on the location of the atresia, resection of the area and an end-to-end anastomosis is carried out, or it may be necessary to perform a gastroenterostomy. In the immediate postoperative period the baby is best nursed in an incubator where the temperature, humidity and oxygen inflow (if required) can be easily regulated and the baby's condition readily observed. Aspiration of the stomach contents should be continued at intervals and when the amount of aspirate is negligible and bowel sounds have returned then oral feeding may be commenced. The baby should be offered water in a bottle for the first few feeds, and if this is not vomited and the amount of aspirate does not increase then milk feeds may be introduced; it would be preferable for breast milk to be given at this stage even if the baby is weaned to cow's milk before discharge home. When feeding is progressing well then the infusion should be discontinued. Observations of the temperature and pulse and respiratory rates together with colour are important, and accurate records should be kept. It should be noted when the baby passes urine, and the colour and frequency of the stools passed should be recorded. Abdominal sutures will be removed about the eighth post-operative day. Handling and toilet care should be kept to the minimum (*see* page 238). Prognosis is good for the full term infant and where no complications have occurred, but the situation is less favourable where there is prematurity and possibly other malformations.

Diverticula

Congenital diverticula occurring in the intestine are more frequently found in the large gut rather than the small, but those in the latter may be either true diverticula where the pouch contains all layers of the wall, or false, where only the mucosa and not the muscle layer herniates. True diverticula are usually found in the upper small intestine and include duodenal and Meckel's diverticulum. False diverticula mainly occur in the jejunum and remain symptomless, just occasionally contributing to the malabsorption syndrome.

Meckel's diverticulum

This congenital anomaly occurs due to a persistent remnant which connects the ileum to the umbilicus during early fetal development. In the majority of instances it does not give rise to symptoms, but occasionally the gut becomes inflamed giving the appearance of appendicitis. Later, this may be responsible for volvulus occurring, or it may be the starting point of intussusception (*see* Chapter 12), for which surgery will be necessary. A loop of gut present in the base of the umbilical cord may prevent separation of the cord within a few days of birth; although this is a rare anomaly the midwife should bear this possibility in mind and refer the baby to the doctor for investigation rather than apply a further clamp or ligature when the cord fails to shrink and separate.

TRAUMA

Foreign bodies

Children between the ages of one and four years are prone to swallowing small beads, buttons, plastic toys etc. and the majority of these objects pass uneventfully through the whole gastro-intestinal tract. If this fails to occur then it is the curves of the duodenum which usually prove an obstacle to their smooth passage. At first, symptoms are not present, but in time the area becomes oedematous and eventually this may progress to ulceration and perforation of the gut wall. The whole of the gastrointestinal tract should be X-rayed, and this repeated at frequent intervals especially in the case of a pointed object traversing the gut. Surgical removal of the foreign body should be undertaken for any object that remains stationary for seven days.

MALABSORPTION SYNDROME

This term is used collectively for a number of conditions resulting from abnormal absorption of nutrients in the gut. Since the bulk of foodstuffs are absorbed during their passage through the small intestine then this area is the most likely to be affected, although once a particular disease becomes established it may involve a greater area of gut mucosa and spread into the large intestine. This syndrome may originate from abnormalities in the lumen of the gut which may affect the production of enzymes, their ability to mix with the foodstuffs or the action of the commensal bacteria; or it may result from alteration in the structure of the intestinal wall, such as the lack of villi demonstrated in coeliac disease. Finally, it may originate from influences outside of the gut as a complication of such systemic conditions as polyarteritis nodosa, severe skin lesions or as a result of chemotherapy, especially the anticoagulant drug phenindione. Characteristically, malabsorption syndrome has three main features: (1) nutritional abnormality; (2) diarrhoea, with or without steatorrhoea; and (3) abdominal discomfort.

Nutritional abnormality

Although in the majority of these diseases diarrhoea with bulky pale stools is a common feature it is not only fat that is poorly absorbed from the diet; all essential nutrients may be affected. The inability to absorb carbohydrate may be demonstrated by the xylose test (*see* page 176) and also in the flat curve observed following a glucose tolerance test. Protein absorption is not so commonly affected except at times of exacerbation of the condition. Vitamins are poorly absorbed and because of this, certain features of the syndrome are noted, namely lack of vitamin B leading to stomatitis, glossitis and skin lesions; vitamin D deficiency contributing to osteomalacia and possibly bony fractures, and lack of vitamin B_{12} manifesting itself in both macrocytic and megaloblastic anaemia. Lack of absorption of electrolytes where the blood levels of calcium, phosphorus, chloride, sodium and potassium are particularly low is without doubt one of the causes of the muscle weakness and general fatigue which is characteristic of these diseases. The appetite is usually good.

Diarrhoea and steatorrhoea

Diarrhoea may persist in a number of patients but in some may only occur for a few days on two or three occasions each year. In others, bowel habits may be normal, or they may even complain of constipation. If steatorrhoea is present then the stools are large, bulky, pale and often frothy in appearance.

Abdominal discomfort

Abdominal pain is a feature of this syndrome and is due to distension, although epigastric pain may be complained of and resemble that of peptic ulceration. It is usual for the patient to pass large quantities of flatus.

Other clinical features which may be observed include a shiny pigmented skin lacking in hair, hypotension, oedema and skin haemorrhages (possibly due to lack of vitamin K). The patient may give a history of some of these features occurring over a number of years, with a gradual loss of weight, fatigue and deterioration in general health. Admission to hospital should be advised so that a number of tests may be carried out and a specific diagnosis made. The patient may feel reasonably well and not wish to remain in hospital, but it is essential their cooperation be obtained at the outset so that accurate preparations can be made for the tests and therefore a reliable result obtained.

Investigations

Investigations will include: *Haematology*—iron, folic acid and vitamin B_{12} uptake tests; and *Biochemistry*—blood levels particularly of calcium ions, phosphorus, phosphate and prothrombin time.

Absorption tests (1) The amount of faecal fat present is estimated by collecting the total stools passed during three days following the administration of 100 g fat daily in the diet for three days; the total amount of fat present is divided by three. If more than 6 g fat is excreted in twenty-four hours then a diagnosis of steatorrhoea is made.

(2) Xylose test. This synthetic sugar is almost completely absorbed by the jejunum in normal health. 25 g xylose is given in the morning after the patient has starved overnight. All urine passed during the next five hours is collected and the xylose content estimated, similarly a blood sample is taken after one and a half hours.

(3) Schilling test. Radioactive cobalt is used to ascertain the absorption of vitamin B_{12} in the investigation of pernicious anaemia (*see* page 290).

Radiological investigations will include observations of the gut following a barium meal and follow through, and also X-raying of the whole skeleton to demonstrate possible bony changes. Following X-ray of the gut, areas of stricture may be seen which are characteristic of Crohn's disease (regional ileitis, or more correctly regional enteritis as it may affect any part of the gastrointestinal tract).

Biopsy of the jejunum with the aid of a Crosby capsule will indicate the mucosal changes which may have occurred, and give a precise diagnosis for such conditions as coeliac disease. Following a period of starvation the patient swallows a tube to which is attached a small capsule (Crosby). When its presence in the jejunum has been confirmed by X-ray, aspiration of the tube will cause the nearest area of mucosa to be sucked to the capsule and a tiny blade severs it from the wall. The tube complete with specimen may then be removed.

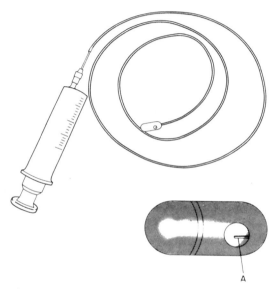

Fig. 51. *Crosby capsule. The blade is shown at 'A'.*

Other tests which may be carried out include a bacteriological estimation and analysis of the bile salt content. When the results of these various tests are known then a precise diagnosis can be made and treatment instigated. Irrespective of the diagnosis the patient will probably be given a low fat diet, and an attempt made to correct all deficiencies by the administration of iron, folic acid, vitamins B_{12} and D, and calcium. Specific treatment will be discussed with each condition.

Coeliac disease in children

This condition usually shows itself once the child has become established on mixed feeding, and symptoms may present anytime from then until about two years of age. Diarrhoea, loss of weight, vomiting and irritability are common, and without treatment complications of rickets, anaemia, oedema and frequent intercurrent infections are likely to occur. The condition may well continue on into adult life. Examination of the intestinal mucosa shows an absence of villi, giving a virtually flat appearance. It has been shown that foods prepared from rye and wheat flour cause an exacerbation of this condition because they contain the protein, gluten; if gluten can be removed entirely from the diet then symptoms will disappear and the small intestine return to normal functioning after a few weeks. The main problem associated with this treatment is that flour containing gluten is used in the preparation of so many foodstuffs that great care and supervision must be exercised on the part of the parents to see that a gluten-containing food is not eaten by the child. Certain bakery firms do now supply gluten-free flour for cooking and also biscuits and ready-made cakes. Gluten is present in a wide range of foodstuffs and must be entirely avoided; these include such children's favourites as baked beans, chocolate, cream, custard, ice cream, canned meats and potato crisps to mention but a few. The prognosis following early diagnosis and strict adherence to a gluten-free diet is excellent; prior to finding the cause of coeliac disease many children died at a very young age.

Coeliac disease in adults (*Idiopathic steatorrhoea*)

This is a similar condition to that found in children, but may be diagnosed after investigation of symptoms which may suggest other conditions. Patients may complain of tetany, loss of weight and glossitis, and may be found to have severe anaemia, diarrhoea and dyspepsia similar to that experienced by the patient with peptic ulceration. Skeletal changes are frequently noted, and pain may be experienced due to osteomalacia. Poor absorption and diarrhoea may give rise to electrolyte disturbance. Investigations should resemble those described for children, and similar changes in the intestinal mucosa will be noted. Hypotension and skin pigmentation occur (also characteristic of Addison's disease) but if there is persistent diarrhoea the physician should undertake full investigation of the gastrointestinal tract as this is suggestive of adult coeliac disease. Malignancy in the tract must also be considered as this may accompany coeliac disease in adults. Treatment of adults should be along the same lines as indicated for children, including the treatment of all associated conditions such as anaemia.

Tropical sprue

This is a condition which mainly affects middle-aged adults who have spent many years in the tropics. The features of tropical sprue closely resemble those of coeliac disease, but examination of the jejunum following biopsy will show only partial atrophy of the villi, and this is due to lack of vitamin B_{12} and not the presence of gluten in the diet. If the patient responds to treatment with a gluten-free diet then the correct diagnosis would have been adult coeliac disease. Tropical sprue runs a fairly consistent course of exacerbations and periods of remission. Treatment is effected by the administration of vitamin B_{12} by injection, folic acid by mouth and a course of an antibiotic such as tetracycline 500 mg four times a day for several months. During an acute phase dehydration and electrolyte imbalance may need to be corrected by giving the patient an intravenous infusion. Following treatment improvement in the state of the intestinal villi will be noted.

Regional enteritis (*Crohn's disease*)

Although the terminal ileum and caecum are more often affected in this condition it can occur at any level of the gastrointestinal tract and is therefore more correctly called regional enteritis. Crohn's disease is a chronic condition persisting throughout the patient's life usually starting in the early twenties; it affects men more than women, but appears not to be related to race or social class.

Aetiology is unknown but various theories have been put forward including psychosomatic disorders, but there is no real foundation for this theory, or that it is an autoimmune disease. The onset of the condition is slow, intermittent attacks of diarrhoea occurring over a period of several months, until colicky abdominal pain is experienced and relieved by the diarrhoea. There is an associated anaemia, pyrexia, weight loss and possibly psychological disturbances such as depression. Some patients experience an acute attack with nausea and vomiting, and pain which resembles that of appendicitis which may lead the surgeon to perform an exploratory laparotomy and thus arrive at a diagnosis.

Characteristically the terminal ileum appears thickened, oedematous and red, with a thick mesentery and enlarged lymph nodes, the lumen of the gut being considerably reduced. The mucosa becomes ulcerated in patches and with the non-affected areas in between gives a blotchy appearance. Lesions may become adherent to neighbouring coils of gut and fistulae occur between them and it is not uncommon for a fistula to track down and open into the perineum. An ischio-rectal abscess or fistula-in-ano should alert the doctor to the possibility of the presence of Crohn's disease. Stenosis of the affected ileum will show on an X-ray when a barium meal and follow through has been carried out. Laparotomy may also be necessary.

Treatment may be either medical, surgical or a combination of both. The aim of medical treatment is to improve the nutrition of the patient by giving a high calorie and high protein diet, low in roughage and with additional vitamins. Anaemia will require treatment. In the acute febrile stage a broad spectrum antibiotic should be given, and this may be combined with the administration of a corticosteroid such as prednisolone. After the acute phase has passed this latter drug may be considerably reduced to the level of a maintenance dose. Occasionally corticosteroids are combined with a sulphonamide such as sulphasalazine. The use of immunosuppressive drugs such as azathioprine may sometimes be indicated. Surgical treatment consists of resection of that part of the gut which is involved, although variation as to the exact technique is found from one surgeon to another. On the whole the minimum of gut is removed, and the formation of blind loops avoided as these predispose to the complications of the malabsorption syndrome; abscess formation and fistulae. It must also be expected that absorption of vitamin B_{12} will be impaired following operation, and this should be supplemented by intramuscular injections at regular intervals. Surgery relieves rather than cures this condition, and recurrence is common. Crohn's disease may affect the colon, and a description of this is included in the next chapter.

Other causes of malabsorption syndrome

Other causes of malabsorption syndrome include lack of bile as found in obstructive jaundice, or lack of pancreatic enzymes associated with carcinoma of the head of the pancreas, following surgery of the gastrointestinal tract such as a large resection of the small gut or partial gastrectomy, and in association with other generalized diseases and skin conditions. Finally, infestations with intestinal parasites may also cause this situation to arise.

INFLAMMATORY AND INFECTIVE CONDITIONS

Tuberculous enteritis

This is an uncommon condition and may present in either a primary or secondary form.

Primary tuberculosis is usually bovine, acquired by drinking infected milk. Incidence of this disease is almost entirely confined to countries where strict control over cattle and milk supplies is not exercised. Enlargement of the mesenteric lymph nodes will be seen on X-ray. Treatment is by antituberculous chemotherapy.

Secondary tuberculosis may result from the swallowing of infected sputum in a patient with an active pulmonary lesion. Similar X-ray appearances will be noted to those seen in the primary condition and treatment will follow a similar pattern. Malabsorption may occur as a complication.

Typhoid fever

Infection in the gut by the *Salmonella* organisms may be of a mild variety causing food poisoning or a more severe form which causes typhoid fever. This condition occurs as a result of infection by *Salmonella typhi* which enters the gastrointestinal tract by ingestion of infected food or fluid. The organisms pass into the small intestine where they enter the lymphoid follicles having penetrated the wall, and are carried to the mesenteric lymph nodes and Peyer's patches. Proliferation of organisms occurs and they are subsequently conveyed through the lymphatics to the thoracic duct and so into the systemic circulation. A positive blood culture is obtainable during the first week of the disease. Now that the bacilli have reached the blood stream they are conveyed to the liver, spleen, lungs and bone marrow and will be passed to the gall bladder in the bile which becomes heavily infected. It is worth noting that some patients continue to harbour the organism long after clinical signs of the disease have disappeared, the gall bladder continually excreting organisms into the gut which are passed in the faeces. This carrier state may be difficult to treat and often requires a cholecystectomy to be performed. Outbreaks of this disease, the tracing of the source of infection and the long-term follow up of potential carriers has improved considerably during this century due to better sanitation, sewage disposal, improved water supplies and supervision of establishments where food is prepared and sold.

The typical course of this disease is of the gradual onset of malaise, headache and pyrexia following an incubation period which varies from ten to thirty days. Anorexia, nausea and vomiting may be present in the early stages and epistaxis is common. During the second week the pyrexia is sustained, a macular rash appears on the trunk; the crops of 'rose spots' lasting two or three days. Abdominal distension is present and severe diarrhoea occurs, the stools being loose and green containing occult blood. General aches and pains are complained of, and delirium may be present. Necrosis of Peyer's patches may occur at this time, followed by ulceration in the third week of the disease when sloughing of the intestinal wall may result in severe haemorrhage. Organisms are present in large numbers in the stools during the second week and may also be isolated from the urine. Towards the end of the third week the patient may die from a general toxaemia, or gradual improvement in the condition may take place with a lessening of all symptoms. Ideally, diagnosis should be made as early as possible and with the administration of an antibiotic such as chloramphenicol rapid recovery should take place and the severe symptoms of the second and third week should not occur. Chloramphenicol 500 mg four times a day should be continued for about ten days, and although it is known to cause blood dyscrasias its use is justified in the treatment of this particular disease with a known high mortality rate. Diagnosis can be assisted by isolating the organism by blood culture or from the stools or urine, or by demonstrating the presence of agglutinins to *Salmonella typhi* by the Widal test where a titre of over 1 in 50 is regarded as positive. Besides chemotherapy, treatment of dehydration, electrolyte balance and possible blood transfusion if haemorrhage has occurred will be necessary.

Nursing care of this ill person will be directed to maintaining the comfort of a febrile patient with particular attention to the skin and mouth; incontinence of faeces may occur in the delirious state. The patient must be isolated and all excreta rendered harmless by means of a disinfectant before disposal. Gowns and possibly gloves should be worn when attending to the patient. Careful observations should be made and recorded; also any change in the general condition. The patient is not discharged until the stools and urine are bacteriologically clear.

Paratyphoid fever

This is caused by one of the *Salmonella paratyphi* organisms either A, B or C, and resembles typhoid fever in its appearance and course, although in all respects it is much less severe. Diagnosis and treatment is the same as that described for *Salmonella typhi*.

NEOPLASTIC CONDITIONS

Malignant tumours are a rare occurrence in the small intestine and if they do occur are likely to be lymphosarcomas. Growth of the neoplasm will eventually reduce the lumen of the gut, but obstruction is a very late feature of the condition as the contents are still fluid as they pass on into the large intestine. It is probable that metastases will already be present by the time the primary lesion is diagnosed and thus the prognosis on the whole is poor.

CHAPTER 9

The Large Intestine

The large intestine is greater in diameter than the small intestine, being wider at the caecum and gradually tapering towards the rectum. The mucosa differs from that of the small intestine in that it possesses no villi but has a much greater number of goblet cells and therefore can produce quantities of mucus; this lubricates the faeces and assists in their passage along the gut. The proximal part of the colon contains lymph nodules along the wall, especially in the appendix. The longitudinal muscle arrangement is of three strands forming an incomplete covering and thus allowing the circular fibres and mucosa to sacculate between the strands, the taenia coli. When fully distended the large intestine has a capacity of just less than two litres.

Movements of the large intestine

Chyme is propelled into the large intestine in periodic bursts as the ileo-caecal valve opens momentarily, but after this the contents move slowly through the large gut, the ascending and transverse colons filling passively aided only by minimal peristalsis. The rate of progress through the large intestine varies considerably from one individual to another, and also regarding the composition of the contents, but it is known that a barium meal which takes about four hours to reach the large intestine will take a further two hours to

185

pass through the ascending colon to the hepatic flexure, a further three hours to the splenic flexure and another three hours to reach the pelvic colon. About 75% of a barium meal (which passes more quickly through the gut than food residues) will have been expelled by seventy-two hours, but the remainder may take four to five days. During this time the faeces are continually being mixed by segmentation which occurs due to action of the gut wall. Three or four times a day a massive peristaltic movement drives the large gut contents towards the rectosigmoid junction where the faeces are held. The nerve supply to the proximal colon is by the vagus nerves, and to the distal colon by other parasympathetic fibres passing out from the spinal cord with the second, third and fourth sacral nerves to join the hypogastric plexus before ennervating the rectum and internal anal sphincter. The external sphincter of striated muscle is under voluntary control by the action of the pudendal nerve.

Defaecation

One of the large peristaltic waves which occurs each day will propel faeces into the rectum where a sensation of fullness will be experienced initiating a desire to defaecate; this is likely to follow shortly after taking a meal as the stomach fills. The mucosa will become red and secrete more mucus. The act of defaecation starts with the voluntary contraction of the muscles of the abdominal wall and the diaphragm. With the breath being held the intra-abdominal pressures rises; simultaneously, there is a relaxation of the anal sphincters accompanied by powerful peristaltic movements on the part of the gut to convey the contents through the rectum and anal canal. These movements are assisted by the contraction of the levator ani muscles which pull the anal canal upwards and over the descending mass of faeces. Normally defaecation empties the sigmoid descending colon of faeces, but if strong aperients are taken then the whole of the large bowel may empty and take two or three days to refill. The habitual use of purgatives will lead to electrolyte loss, especially potassium. If defaecation is delayed then the sensation gradually fades and during the increased time that the faeces remain in the colon more water is absorbed and constipation results. The number of times each day or week that defaecation takes place will vary considerably but will be the accepted pattern for each individual. One person may normally empty the bowel twice a day whereas another only three times per week, and both remain in good health. Severe injury to the spinal cord above the level of the sacral region removes the voluntary control over defaecation but allows a reflex action to continue; this results in complete expulsion of faeces but the individual is unaware of it taking place and is unable to control the act. Sudden distension of the rectum causes a desire to pass flatus; as the distension is less than that caused by the presence of faeces distinction between the two sensations is possible, the sphincters are then relaxed to allow air to pass out.

Formation of the faeces

About 350 g of chyme enters the large intestine daily and from this a considerable volume of water is reabsorbed mainly by the caecum and ascending colon, so that on average 100 g of actual faeces are produced each day. Absorption includes not only water but sodium chloride, anaesthetic drugs and some steroids, whilst proteins, fats and sugars are not well absorbed by the large gut. By the end of their thirty-six hour stay in the large intestine the faeces will have a pH of about 7·5 and contain:

60–80% water;

a little undigested or unabsorbed foodstuff, mainly cellulose, skins and seeds of fruit;

bile and other secretions such as mucus, leucocytes and desquamated epithelium;

10–20% inorganic matter mainly of calcium and phosphates, bacteria.

The colour of the faeces is due to stercobilin formed from bile pigments, but this may be changed to black as a result of the presence of altered blood, or a clay colour when there is lack of bile. The characteristic odour is partly due to the fermentation of carbohydrate and also to the presence of skatole and indole, two end-products of the breakdown of an amino acid, tryptophane which are absorbed and detoxified by the liver. Cellulose gives bulk to the faeces and thereby stimulates peristalsis; this factor is the basis of giving roughage in the diet to speed the movement of faeces through the bowel and therefore reduce the amount of water absorbed. The amount of faeces formed is not really related to the dietary intake as they continue to be produced even in conditions of starvation, the quantity being only slightly reduced. As sodium is absorbed by the large bowel so potassium is excreted into the lumen; the patient who experiences intestinal hurry resulting in diarrhoea will lose both sodium and potassium and suffer from the effects of their depletion; this can also occur after repeated colonic irrigations. A study of the faeces can be made by the use of a marker such as radioactive chromium (^{51}Cr) which is not absorbed and can be recovered from the faeces.

Bacteria of the gut

In the newborn infant the gut contents are semifluid in consistency and greenish-black in colour; this meconium is sterile but after a few days organisms acquired from the mother's vagina quickly multiply. A large number of organisms are non-pathogenic and regarded as normal inhabitants of the gut (commensals); they ferment carbohydrate producing the gas carbon dioxide. A large part of the gas in the intestine is swallowed atmospheric air, part is reabsorbed and the remainder passed as flatus. Bacteria in the gut are responsible for the synthesis of some vitamins mainly those of the B complex and vitamin K. Normal intestinal organisms influence the activity of the gut as can be observed when the intestinal flora is altered due to the administration of certain anti-biotics which results in the alteration of bowel activity leading to diarrhoea and the passage of large quantities of flatus. Organisms found in the gut of the breast fed baby are mainly lactobacilli, but on weaning there is a change to anaerobic ones, the coliform organisms. Babies which are entirely bottle fed quickly acquire the adult type of intestinal flora. The bacteria form complex relationships between each other and their host, and all are potential pathogens. In the mouth the organisms are mainly the streptococci, especially *Streph. viridans* and *Streph. mutans*: this latter causes dental caries. Some coliform organisms and yeasts may also be present. The stomach is relatively sterile due to the high acidity, but when this becomes neutralized it allows bacteria to pass through unharmed to the small intestine. In the large intestine one-fifth of the wet weight of the faeces is due to bacteria, mainly the non-spore bearing anaerobic organisms such as the bacteroides and enterococci, the latter includes *Strep. faecalis*. These cause little trouble whilst they remain in the gut but are pathogenic if they occur elsewhere in the body. Spore-bearing anaerobic organisms to be found here include the *Clostridia* species which are very resistant and require the autoclaving of contaminated articles. The non-spore bearing aerobic bacteria are less numerous than the anaerobes, but are all potential pathogens. These are the enterobacteria which include the *Escherichia, Klebsiella, Salmonella, Shigella, Proteus* and the related *Pseudomonas* organisms.

Constipation and its treatment

Constipation may be regarded as a state in which no residue of a foodstuff taken on one day has been excreted within the next seventy-two hours. Although acute episodes occur due to the sudden onset of intestinal obstruction or dehydration associated with a severe febrile condition, the majority of cases of constipation are chronic by nature. Chronic constipation may be considered in three main groups:

Dyschezia

This condition results from failure to empty the bowel when the sensation of fullness has been stimulated by contents entering the rectum. If defaecation is delayed then the stimulus passes and does not recur until more faeces enter and distend the rectum. If this situation is allowed to continue the rectum will become more distended until the reflex is not easily stimulated. This type of constipation usually results from faulty habits, mainly because defaecation is delayed because it is inconvenient for some reason. It may also occur in cases of anal fissure where the act of defaecation will cause pain. The situation will not improve with the delay in emptying the bowel as the faeces will become larger and harder in the meantime. General muscular weakness as may be experienced by the elderly and infirm may lead to impaction of faeces in the rectum. The regular use of aperients may cause complete emptying of the colon. Further aperients may be taken because there has been no further bowel action for two or more days, it not being appreciated that the large intestine will take this time to refill.

Treatment is aimed at re-education, both of the patient and the bowel action. A regular daily attempt at defaecation should be made and the stimulus of a full rectum never ignored. The use of aperients should be discouraged but rather the diet should include more roughage and fluids to stimulate quicker peristalsis which can also be aided by the taking of more general exercise. If necessary the addition of bulk substances such as Isogel 5–10 g orally or Normacol 5–10 g orally taken with plenty of water may prove helpful. Senokot is an aperient of vegetable origin which acts by stimulating peristalsis some six or eight hours after administration, the dose is 1–2 tablets and is best taken at night. Impacted faeces may be retained in the rectum and over a period of time will become harder, larger and more difficult to pass. The situation may not be diagnosed as such but rather as one of diarrhoea, as it is possible for the soft faecal matter above to pass round the mass and be excreted, along with excess mucus whose production is stimulated. If the condition is unrelieved then vomiting and abdominal pain may become present. Faecal impaction occurs mainly in the elderly and frail, and sometimes in young children. Treatment is by the slow administration into the rectum of a small quantity (120 ml) of warm olive oil which is allowed to remain for a few hours to soften the mass prior to carrying out a digital removal of the faeces.

Occasionally an enema is required to empty the bowel and this can be either a soap and water solution of 600–1000 ml introduced through a funnel and tubing, or more frequently in these days a disposable type of enema containing about 150 ml of sodium phosphate in a plastic pack which has a short rigid nozzle attached for easy administration. Suppositories may also be used and these both stimulate peristalsis in the rectum and lubricate the faeces, effecting a bowel action after about twenty minutes. Suppositories may be glycerol (glycerine) or bisacodyl (Dulcolax); usually two are given.

Colonic constipation

In this condition stasis results in the slow passage of faeces through the colon, but once the rectum is reached then the reflex stimulation to defaecate is set up and the bowel is emptied normally. This can occur in cases of dehydration and starvation or where there is some organic obstruction to the passage of faeces as may occur with strictures along the wall of the intestine, diverticulosis or the presence of new growths.

Treatment of this condition is mainly that of the underlying cause, the situation improves as the dehydration is corrected or the partial obstruction relieved. Adequate roughage and fluids should also be added to the diet.

Insufficient formation of faeces

Occasionally constipation results from lack of bulk of faeces due to inadequacies of the diet in respect of the amount of food taken especially roughage. There is no delay in the passage of faeces through the large intestine until the pelvic colon is reached, but the lack of bulk fails to distend the gut and stimulate the normal sensation of fullness. Treatment is mainly dietary, but the addition of bulk substances may be needed.

Diarrhoea

The rapid passage of food through the gut may be due to a number of causes, and is probably best considered as either an acute or chronic condition, the former resulting from ingestion of organisms or their toxins, chemical poisons or an overdose of an aperient.

Acute diarrhoea

1. Due to organisms

Acute diarrhoea is mainly the result of gastrointestinal infection, variation is noted as to the causative organism and the country of origin and the time of year that attacks occur. Infection will often be due to *Shigella* organisms (the bacillary type as opposed to the amoebic type of dysentery) of which *Sh. sonnei* is the most frequent cause of outbreaks of diarrhoea in institutions in this country. it is not a severe disease but one that is readily spread by contamination of toilet seats, door handles etc., and which leads to contamination of foodstuffs. *Salmonella* organisms of which there are several hundred species are also responsible for outbreaks of diarrhoea, and it is often due to *S. typhimurium,* an organism which forms part of the normal bacterial flora in animals such as pigs and chickens. The organism is acquired by humans who eat poultry that has not been completely thawed before cooking or from uncooked foods such as salads prepared on the same work surface as infected meat. An acute attack of diarrhoea usually starts twenty-four hours after ingestion of the organisms and may last a few days. A form of diarrhoea with a rapid onset of only four or more hours after ingestion is likely to be the result of *Clostridium welchii* infection. This organism may be present in human and animal faeces and in dirt and dust. It is a very resistant organism producing spores, some of which are not killed by cooking. As the meat cools, the spores germinate and then usually the meat is only reheated to a palatable temperature which is insufficient to kill the organisms. This situation may arise where a large joint of meat has cooled slowly and not been immediately refrigerated; prevention is by cooking meat in small quantities and cooling rapidly.

A considerable number of outbreaks of diarrhoea are of unknown aetiology, but these may be due to viruses. The enterovirus group primarily inhabit the human intestine but may be found in the respiratory tract as well. Infection is spread by ingestion and probably flies play a part in the transmission of disease. This group of viruses include those responsible for poliomyelitis, the Coxsackie viruses which cause a wide range of conditions from meningitis to myocarditis and the common cold; and also the ECHO viruses which cause febrile conditions and attacks of diarrhoea. Pathogenic *E. coli* are responsible for disease occurring in babies and young children which gives rise to diarrhoea which can spread readily to the occupants of a paediatric ward or nursery; or the adult form which may well be one cause of travellers diarrhoea. The source of both types of infection is human.

Profuse diarrhoea is a feature of cholera, caused by the *Vibrio cholerae*. This is a human parasite whose location is entirely restricted to the intestine. It may be spread from one person to another by direct contact or through faecal contamination of drinking water when it is likely to cause a major outbreak of the disease. Frequent watery stools are passed ('rice water' stools) which causes severe dehydration to the patient and may lead to death if untreated. Immunization may be given in the form of a vaccine which is effective for six months.

2. Due to bacterial toxins

An acute form of diarrhoea may be due to the ingestion of bacterial toxins, a situation where the actual organism plays no part in affecting the patient. One of the most likely causes is diarrhoea due to the toxin of *Staph. aureus,* the food having become contaminated from an infected skin lesion on any person concerned with the preparation of the meal. Onset of symptoms is rapid, usually vomiting occurs first followed by diarrhoea with abdominal pain. The patient usually feels very ill for several hours but is much improved the following day.

Although food poisoning due to *Clostridium welchii* was considered under the previous heading, it is possible that this organism also produces a toxin which may be responsible for attacks of diarrhoea; certainly one of its relatives, *Clostridium botulinum* produces a toxin which may be found in contaminated meat, fish and vegetables especially if the foodstuffs have been subjected to canning. Fortunately this form of food poisoning is uncommon as it is particularly lethal as regards the outcome.

Diagnosis and treatment of acute diarrhoea

Culture of the faeces to isolate the organism is necessary and as this takes two to three days to complete in many instances symptoms have subsided by the time the result is known. The *Entamoeba* organisms are large and motile, and can be seen under the microscope provided the specimen of stool is fresh and warm, it is therefore imperative that the specimen is conveyed to the laboratory with urgency as soon as it has been obtained. The history of the outbreak of diarrhoea will often give clues as to the cause, then further investigation of foodstuffs and kitchen staff, water supply and sanitary arrangements will need to be made.

In general, the treatment of diarrhoea (except that due to cholera) is mainly to replace lost body fluid. There are few indications for the administration of antibiotics except in outbreaks of gastroenteritis amongst the newborn or to ill persons who are in hospital for the treatment of some unrelated condition. Sugar in moderation should be added to the oral fluids. Foods containing a high fat content should be avoided whilst diarrhoea persists, but as soon as possible a normal diet should be resumed. As the correction of dehydration is of such importance the intravenous route will be used for babies and ill adults. Besides treating the condition the nurse must constantly be aware of the dangers of spread of the infection, the patient should be isolated, stools decontaminated before disposal, all feeding utensils kept separately or sterilized after use, and strict adherence to personal hygiene and hand washing carried out.

The treatment of cholera follows the same principles except that a greater fluid intake will be necessary by the intravenous route as it is possible for the patient to lose as much as twenty litres of body fluid daily in the watery stools. Administration of tetracycline shortens the duration of the illness. Outbreaks of cholera may well result from contamination of a town's water supply by infected sewage, and so extensive investigations will need to be conducted.

Chronic diarrhoea

Chronic diarrhoea may be associated with other gastrointestinal disturbances such as the malabsorption syndrome, carcinoma, pancreatic conditions or follow operations on the stomach such as partial gastrectomy. In the latter case advice regarding the diet, and the size and temperature of meals may be all that is necessary to bring about an improvement in the situation. For the other conditions named, treatment is aimed at the underlying cause and when improvement is noted there is often a reduction in the attacks of diarrhoea.

Diarrhoea due to non-gastrointestinal causes

Occasionally diarrhoea is a feature of conditions which are not directly related to the gastrointestinal tract. These include psychosomatic disorders which may be responsible for irritable colon, or diarrhoea resulting from allergy to certain foods or drugs, endocrine and metabolic disorders, and diarrhoea due to vitamin deficiency and radiation.

CONGENITAL ANOMALIES

A number of congenital anomalies occur in the large gut, including Hirschsprung's disease, volvulus, diverticula and imperforate anus.

Hirschsprung's disease

This is due to lack of innervation of part of the large intestine where there is an absence of the ganglia of both Auerbach's and Meissner's plexus which are responsible for initiating peristaltic movements of the gut wall; therefore chronic constipation is the chief feature of this condition.

Hirschsprung's disease shows a familial incidence. The lack of co-ordinated peristalsis gives rise to periods of alternating diarrhoea and constipation which results in failure to thrive on the part of the child. The abdomen becomes distended and visible peristalsis may

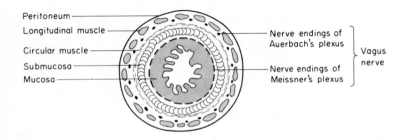

Fig. 52. *Diagrammatic cross-section of gut wall.*

be noted, together with increased bowel sounds. Diagnosis may be made in the immediate neonatal period when there is delay in the passage of meconium and subsequent stools, or it may not be made until the baby is older and obviously has constipation of a chronic type. Diagnosis is assisted by a plain X-ray of the abdomen which shows the presence of fluid levels, or if barium is introduced into the gut then a narrowed segment is seen. For the neonate as a temporary measure the treatment is to raise a colostomy in an unaffected segment of gut until further permanent surgery can be undertaken when the baby is older. Later, the affected length of gut is resected and an end to end anastomosis carried out. The prognosis of this operation is directly related to the extent of the aganglionic segment of bowel which needs to be removed.

A complication of Hirschsprung's disease is enterocolitis, a condition which can quickly prove fatal. Large quantities of fluids and electrolytes are lost into the lumen of the gut, together with those lost from the accompanying diarrhoea and vomiting. Treatment is by replacement of fluids and electrolytes by the intravenous route and the administration of a broad spectrum antibiotic.

Volvulus

Volvulus may occur in the neonatal period due to abnormalities of the supporting mesentery of the gut. This condition will give rise to intestinal obstruction and is considered along with other congenital causes in Chapter 12.

Imperforate anus

This is among the most common of congenital malformations, occurring about 1 in 1000 births. It is a collective term for several anomalies present in the rectum and anal canal which probably arise from arrested development in this area in the six to twelve week old fetus. About one-sixth of babies with this malformation also have other congenital defects which include hydronephrosis, malformed spine and heart anomalies. A fistula may also develop between the rectum and perineum, the vagina or urinary tract. The blind end of the gut may be either 'high' at the anorectal junction, or 'low' at the anal outlet; some 50% of the former have a lumbosacral spine defect which shows on X-ray and there is a high incidence of renal tract abnormalities for which an intravenous pyelogram should be carried out. In the majority of babies a dimple is present at the normal site of the anus, and the midwife should investigate this by attempting the careful introduction of a well lubricated rectal thermometer when carrying out the initial examination of the baby shortly after birth. Force should never be used and if in any doubt the baby must be referred urgently to the doctor. If the abnormality is of the 'low' type then this can usually be dealt with in the neonatal period, or the surgeon may prefer immediately to raise a colostomy and carry out reconstructive surgery later. Raising a colostomy is also indicated for the 'high' variety, and when the baby is about six to nine months old an abdominoperineal operation is performed aimed at bringing the rectum to the surface of the perineum; the success rate for this operation is that about 75% of children operated on will have satisfactory anal function.

INFLAMMATORY AND INFECTIVE CONDITIONS

Inflammation can occur at any level of the gastrointestinal tract but perhaps those conditions which are chronic and cause greatest distress to the patient are the ones associated with the large intestine. These include: diverticulitis, appendicitis, ulcerative colitis, Crohn's disease and fistula-in-ano.

Diverticulitis

Diverticula occur in both the small and large intestine and originate as either true or false; the former were discussed in the chapter on the small intestine as these pouches contain all layers of the gut wall and are true congenital anomalies such as Meckel's diverticulum. The false diverticula are formed of the gut mucosa only which herniates through a congenital weakness of the large gut wall between the bands of the taenia coli mainly in the sigmoid colon. This situation rarely gives rise to problems before the age of fifty years when it affects about 20% of people. Together, the diverticula constitute the condition of diverticulosis, and only at intervals do these pouches become inflamed to be then termed diverticulitis. The cause of diverticulosis is thought to be due to a high intraluminal pressure which may originate from a relatively low residue diet; the condition may be symptomless or may produce disturbances in bowel habits or lead to acute diverticulitis following the impaction of a faecolith in a diverticulum. The patient usually experiences sudden severe lower and left sided abdominal pain, accompanied by pyrexia, a raised pulse rate and leucocytosis is noted on blood film examination. The findings are usually sufficient to make a diagnosis possible, but if not a barium enema may show the diverticula or a block in the sigmoid colon.

The treatment of acute inflammation is to encourage rest in bed and relief of the pain with a suitable analgesic such as pethidine hydrochloride. Fluids only should be given by mouth and if the intake is insufficient they may need to be given intravenously. A broad spectrum antibiotic such as ampicillin will be prescribed. When the acute condition has subsided the patient should be encouraged to resume a normal diet with a high roughage content, bulk in the gut stimulates peristalsis and discourages inflammatory reactions. Complications may occur with acute diverticulitis; these include the formation of a pericolic abscess which if not drained immediately may lead to fistula formation between it and the abdominal wall or the perineum (ischio-rectal abscess); a temporary colostomy is raised in order to rest the colon. Perforation of the colon leading to a general peritonitis may occur. This is best treated by a temporary colostomy or resection of the affected part of the gut and anastomosis. Purulent material may enter the portal system and be conveyed to the liver later giving rise to portal pyaemia which is treated by antibiotics.

Diverticulosis may be the cause of profuse rectal bleeding, particularly in the middle aged and elderly patient which will result in severe anaemia. Blood transfusion is indicated as treatment particularly as further haemorrhage may occur after several months. On the whole, diverticulosis is treated by attention to the diet in order to prevent diverticulitis occurring rather than resecting a large area of affected gut and performing an end to end anastomosis. This condition has been found not to predispose to carcinoma of the colon, but both conditions may be present alongside one another.

Appendicitis

This inflammatory condition may occur in either sex at almost any time of life, although it is unusual to present before the age of two years. Appendicitis is more common in western civilization and statistics show there to be a higher incidence amongst the middle and upper social classes; several theories have been put forward to explain this including the fact that the diet of the least financially endowed is likely to contain more vegetable and cellulose products than meat, although this is by no means the entire solution to the problem.

Inflammation of the appendix may be broadly divided into two groups, acute and chronic, the former again being divided into that caused by obstruction, or infection which is blood-borne. Obstruction of the appendix is regarded as the most serious form as there is no escape route for the appendix contents except through the wall. This type is more likely to progress to gangrene of the appendix, rupture and general peritonitis. In the blood-borne infective (catarrhal) type, drainage is still possible back into the caecum and therefore perforation is unlikely.

Acute obstructive appendicitis

The impacted faecolith which obstructs the lumen of the appendix may be a nut or seed, and very occasionally this becomes calcified. The appendix mucosa is stimulated to secrete even more mucus which adds to the distension in the organ and drives the bacteria into and through the wall to the adjoining tissues such as the loops of small gut or the surrounding peritoneum; these bacteria set up an acute inflammatory reaction which may cause thrombosis of the appendicular artery which predisposes to gangrene and perforation of the appendix. Should these changes occur slowly then there is more likelihood of the infection being localized by the sealing off of the appendix by the formation of adhesions in the surrounding omentum resulting in an appendix abscess, otherwise a more widespread infection will occur leading to general peritonitis. An appendix abscess should be drained as this too may rupture into the peritoneal cavity.

The patient will give a history of colicky type central abdominal pain starting a few hours earlier and which then migrates to the right iliac fossa becoming continuous and more intense in character. The patient feels nauseated and may vomit. On examination there is tenderness and rigidity of the abdomen over McBurney's point (if a line joining the umbilicus to the anterior superior iliac spine is divided into three, then the position where the lateral third joins the medial two-thirds is over the base of the appendix) and the maximum intensity of pain is felt over the appendix. This is not always in the right iliac fossa as the position of the appendix may be pelvic or retrocaecal. If the peritoneum overlying the appendix has

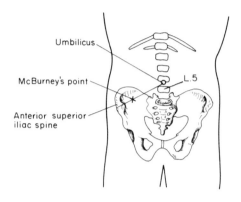

Fig. 53. *McBurney's point.*

become involved in the inflammatory process then sudden withdrawal of the examining hand will cause pain; this is known as rebound tenderness. Observations of the temperature and pulse rate are likely to reveal an increase in both, and blood investigation will show a leucocytosis. In the event of perforation having occurred the abdominal pain and tenderness will be widespread. There will be increasing abdominal distension and an absence of bowel sounds. The temperature and pulse rate will be raised, particularly the latter, and the blood pressure will fall. Atypical cases of acute obstructive appendicitis occur sometimes in the two extremes of life, the very young and the elderly, when there may just be pain in the right iliac fossa and no other symptoms. The danger of this situation is that there may be delay in making a diagnosis which may complicate the treatment.

Treatment

The treatment for this form of appendicitis is mainly surgical, that is removal of the appendix. In certain circumstances the surgeon may prefer to wait until the acute inflammation has subsided before operating as there is an increased mortality with carrying out an appendicectomy at what is judged as the 'wrong' time. The surgeon's aim is to remove the appendix before perforation occurs and for this reason acute pain requires urgent operation, but if an appendix abscess has already formed then some surgeon's prefer to employ conservative treatment. If this is successful the appendix is removed about three months later, or if the abscess is obviously increasing then it must be drained. If the appendix is not removed in the acute stage, then it must be removed when the inflammatory process has subsided, or risk subsequent gangrene and perforation. If peritonitis has occurred then immediate laparotomy is indicated, plus appendicectomy and probably peritoneal drainage; this patient will certainly require restoration of the fluid and electrolyte balance by the intravenous route and the administration of a broad spectrum antibiotic such as ampicillin. The complications of this type of appendicitis are those of local sepsis, pulmonary infection and embolism, along with a fluid and electrolyte imbalance.

Chronic appendicitis

Chronic appendicitis may be due to one of a number of causes which include fibrosis of the appendix following an acute obstructive attack, the lodging of foreign bodies in the appendix, chronic inflammatory reaction of the lymphoid tissue in the appendix wall or the formation of a mucocele, when the contents of the appendix although obstructing its lumen remain sterile. Chronic appendicitis is characterized by dull pain in the right iliac fossa which occasionally gives rise to an acute attack with vomiting.

Treatment

Laparotomy is performed and the appendix removed. Sometimes it looks healthy but most surgeons will remove it in any case to prevent the occurrence of an acute attack. If appendicectomy does not cure the abdominal pain then this is one possible cause which has been eliminated.

Tumours of the appendix

Both benign and malignant tumours of the appendix are rare, of the latter an adenocarcinoma may occur and this is likely to be in an elderly person. On further examination secondary growths are found in the regional lymph nodes and the liver. Surgical treatment consists of hemicolectomy and anastomosis.

Surgical procedures

When the diagnosis of appendicitis is certain the appendix is usually removed through a grid-iron incision as this method of removal carries the lowest mortality rate. An incision is made at right angles to a line joining the anterior superior iliac spine to the umbilicus, the centre of the incision being over McBurney's point. Prior to amputation of the appendix a purse-string suture is put around the caecum through the taenia coli 1·25 cm from the base of the appendix, and following removal of the appendix the stump is

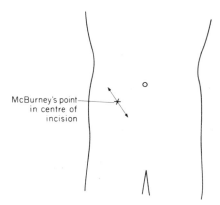

McBurney's point in centre of incision

Fig. 54. *Position of grid iron incision.*

invaginated into the caecum and buried before tying the suture. If diagnosis is uncertain then a lower right paramedian incision is used which enables the surgeon to have access to the pelvic organs or to extend the incision upwards to facilitate surgery of the duodenum.

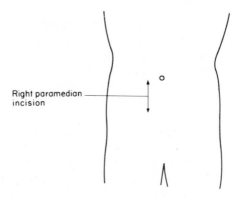

Right paramedian incision

Fig. 55. *Position of paramedian incision.*

Although the approach route to the appendix is different a similar method of removal is employed. Drainage of the operation site is unlikely to be required following removal of an uncomplicated appendix, but where purulent fluid is found in the pelvis or where peritonitis has already intervened then a corrugated type drainage tube is inserted through a stab incision.

Nursing care

The extent of the preparation of the patient for operation depends on the severity of the situation when the patient is admitted and the amount of time available before the patient is taken to the theatre. Where perforation of the appendix is thought to be imminent then the minimum of pre-operative procedures are carried out, the essentials being that the stomach is empty, the heart and lungs are examined and the urine tested and a consent form for operation signed. There may not be time for more than this and dressing the patient in an operation gown and checking that all prostheses are removed. Sometimes operation is delayed for a few hours whilst an intravenous infusion is set up, a nasogastric tube passed, a specimen of blood taken for investigation including electrolyte levels, and a course of antibiotics commenced; this delay enables the nurse to shave the lower abdomen and the pubic hair and to bed bath the patient checking to see that the umbilicus is clean. Observations of temperature and pulse can also be taken at intervals and recorded. For the patient who has been readmitted for appendicectomy some three months after an acute attack then admission to hospital will probably be the day prior to surgery and follow a normal routine as described in Chapter 1.

The post-operative progress of the majority of patients undergoing appendicectomy should be uncomplicated. Following the regaining of consciousness the patient should be sat up well supported by pillows, and allowed to take small quantities of fluids by mouth when required. An injection of pethidine hydrochloride will make the patient feel more comfortable. The day after operation the patient should be encouraged to be up for toilet purposes and given help where necessary. When bowel sounds are heard a light diet may be commenced progressing to a full diet when the patient feels able. Suppositories may be required to encourage a bowel action if this has not occurred by about the end of the third post-operative day. The dressing over the wound may be removed on the day following surgery and the area sprayed with an aerosol. Sutures will be removed on about the seventh day and provided the patient feels well and is mobile he may be discharged home.

Where complications to the appendix have occurred then the post-operative progress is likely to be slower. The stomach contents will require hourly aspiration through the nasogastric tube, and this may need to remain in place for two or three days until the amount of aspirate is almost nil. Fluids will be continued intravenously and small quantities of fluid by mouth only given when bowel sounds are heard, a light diet being commenced when a suitable oral fluid intake is retained. Antibiotics will be continued, and analgesia given as required. It may be several days before the patient is entirely free from abdominal discomfort. The drainage tube will require to be shortened on the two days following operation and provided the amount of drainage is minimal then it can be removed on about the third day. Care should be taken to see that the discharge from the drainage hole does not come into contact with the stitchline. Alternate sutures may be removed on about the eighth and tenth days after operation. During this time the patient should have been encouraged to become mobile again and physiotherapy will have helped in this respect. Provided the patient feels fit he may be allowed home about twelve days after operation.

Conservative treatment

Very occasionally conservative treatment is undertaken, which may be in isolated situations where it would be impossible to move the patient to hospital for operation, or where there has been delay in the patient seeking medical advice and the course of the acute appendicitis has progressed considerably to form an appendix abscess. Conservative treatment should be regarded as a preliminary to surgery, although the actual operation may not be carried out for about three months. The principles of treatment are to rest both the patient as a whole, and the gastrointestinal tract, whilst maintaining very careful observations of the patient's general condition. A nasogastric tube is passed and the stomach contents aspirated at intervals. Water 30 ml hourly is the only fluid allowed by mouth but the patient is kept hydrated by an intravenous infusion. Broad spectrum antibiotics are given, but no analgesics. If the appendix abscess responds to this treatment then the acute pain should soon be replaced by tenderness. The patient may find the local application of heat comforting. Careful recording of the pulse rate taken hourly should be made; the rate should be reduced within twenty four hours if the treatment is successful. A rise in the pulse rate or temperature, more severe pain and an increase in the amount of gastric aspirate or vomiting are an indication to discontinue conservative treatment in favour of immediate surgery. The nurse will be responsible for the observations on the patient, and for keeping the patient as comfortable as possible, paying particular attention to position, toilet and mouth care.

Ulcerative colitis

This disease of the colon is of moderately common occurrence amongst people who live in western civilization, and those who give up a simple nomadic way of life and take up residence in the large cities have also been shown to become similarly affected after a while; why this should be is not clear but it is thought that the differences in food and the psychological stresses of life in a large town may have some bearing on the incidence of the disease. The condition is characterized by inflammation of the mucosa which always starts in the rectum and spreads upwards. In time it may involve the whole colon but rarely passes beyond the ileo-caecal valve into the small intestine. The mucosa becomes hyperaemic and ulcerates. When the condition reaches a chronic phase the mucosa appears flattened and granulation tissue forms as the ulcers heal. Inflammation may spread to the submucosa where abscess formation occurs; these may rupture into the lumen of the colon, and occasionally the colonic wall may perforate. The aetiology of ulcerative colitis remains unknown, but several theories have been put forward and research is directed towards a number of these including that the inflammatory changes may be due to infection, that it is an allergic disease or an autoimmune one since antibodies have been demonstrated, or that nutritional disorders may be responsible although no one dietary constituent has consistently been found to be lacking. Although some people favour psychosomatic factors to be the cause; these are more likely to be responsible for relapses rather than to initiate the condition.

Ulcerative colitis tends to affect young adults more often than at any other age and is more common in women of fifteen to forty-five years. It is likely too that they have a nervous, anxious and perfectionist type of disposition. The patient complains of diarrhoea, as many as twenty or more stools being passed a day which are liquid and contain blood, and may be associated with colicky type abdominal pain. The condition gives rise to systemic effects and will lead to anaemia, loss of weight, muscle weakness and general malaise. In an acute attack there may be severe electrolyte imbalance which could lead to death. Complications of ulcerative colitis may be local, including severe haemorrhage from the colon and abdominal distension, or general, such as arthritis, particularly of the knees and ankles, aphthous ulcers of the mouth, iritis, conjunctivitis and pyoderma, a skin condition in which the multiple bullae present may burst and become secondarily infected.

Diagnosis

There are three main aids to diagnosis:

(1) Sigmoidoscopy. This should always be carried out and will reveal hyperaemia of the mucosa, possibly with a purulent exudate, and if severe the mucosa will be observed to bleed easily.

(2) Barium enema. The X-ray will show a ragged outline to the barium, thus denoting areas of ulceration along the wall.

(3) Bacteriological examination of the faeces. This is to exclude dysentery.

A differential diagnosis must be made to exclude other inflammatory conditions of the colon particularly regional enteritis, the main difference between the two being that the latter affects the submucosa and almost exclusively the small gut and not the large.

Treatment

The treatment of ulcerative colitis can be either medical or surgical, the former often being used to improve the general health of the patient so that they are fit to undergo surgery. In a severe attack the patient should be admitted to hospital where the dehydration can be corrected by giving intravenous fluids, blood can be transfused and a high protein diet given, by the parenteral route if necessary at first. Drugs such as sulphasalazine (Salazopyrin) which is a combination of salicylic acid and sulphonamide may be given in a dose of 4–6 g daily. Corticosteroids may also be used, either systemically in the form of prednisolone, or locally as a Predsol retention enema. Codeine phosphate or dihydrocodeine may be used both as an analgesic and to reduce the motility of the gut; this latter may also be achieved by giving probanthine. After a few days the symptoms should subside and the patient feel better. Therapy can then be continued by the oral route, and the dose of corticosteroids may be gradually reduced until it is finally discontinued. It is no surprise that these patients feel depressed and apathetic at times, particularly as the frequent diarrhoea, or repeated acute attacks necessitating admission to hospital interfere with work, studies, the home and social life. It is for these reasons that many patients prefer to have surgical treatment although this means life with an ileostomy for the remainder of their days.

Indications for operation are mainly a failure to respond to medical treatment or the occurrence of complications, frequent acute attacks, and the knowledge of the tendency to develop carcinoma if the colitis has been present for some long time. The patient can look forward to a normal life expectancy with an ileostomy although the cause of the disease has not necessarily been eliminated. The most usual operative technique is the one-stage proctocolectomy with a permanent ileostomy, although some surgeons favour retaining the rectum and perform an ileo-rectal anastomosis. The procedure for the proctocolectomy is the same as for abdomino-perineal resection of the rectum (see page 222), but if the patient's condition does not allow the perineal dissection then the rectum is closed at the level of the pelvic diaphragm. Prior to operation the patient not only needs to be as fit as possible but also to be psychologically prepared and willing to accept the ileostomy. Great care must be exercised in siting the position of the stoma, as a few millimetres one way or another can make all the difference to the satisfactory fit of the appliance and the subsequent peace of mind and freedom from skin excoriation. Some surgeons require the patient to be up and walking about wearing the ileostomy appliance to make sure that the stoma will be situated in a comfortable position away from bony prominences or previous scars.

Nursing care
The immediate post-operative care will include the care of the

infusion, aspiration of the stomach contents through the nasogastric tube, care of both abdominal and perineal wounds, together with the general observation and basic nursing care. Specific nursing care centres mainly round the ileostomy, and the teaching and supervision of the patient when he starts to look after this for himself. It must be remembered that the contents of the ileum are very fluid and contain digestive enzymes which can cause extensive skin excoriation if the stool is allowed to flow onto the skin. Thus it is essential that a well fitting disposable polythene bag is applied to a double-sided adhesive plaster surrounding the stoma at the conclusion of the operation. The clear polythene affords suitable observation of the colour and texture of the stoma. Within a few weeks the stools will become thicker, and then semisolid after a few months. A protective paste or cream may be applied around the stoma to keep the skin tissues clean and healthy. In many hospitals a trained stomatherapist advises on the care and types of appliances most suited to individual patients and this aspect of the nursing care is dealth with in some detail in Chapter 10.

Regional enteritis

Although regional enteritis more commonly affects the small intestine lesions may be found anywhere along the colon or rectum giving a patchy appearance and the affected areas are often known as skip lesions. Basically, regional enteritis can be distinguished from ulcerative colitis by its pathology, the former affects the submucosa causing multiple granulomata which leads to fibrous thickening and rigidity of all layers of the wall, whilst the latter always starts in the rectum and spreads upwards affecting the superficial mucosa only. Ulcerative colitis is more likely to cause narrowing of the rectum than regional enteritis. This fact can be demonstrated on X-ray following a barium enema when in the latter condition the rectum is seen to dilate fully compared with the stricture-like appearance when ulcerative colitis is present. Perforation of the gut and haemorrhage are unusual occurrences in regional enteritis, although bleeding may accompany the diarrhoea. Regional enteritis in the large gut is more likely to give rise to other complications such as arthritis, aphthous ulceration of the mouth, erythema nodosum and iritis than are found complicating ulcerative colitis, although similar conditions result from both diseases. Treatment of this condition in the large intestine varies: some favour chemotherapy using corticosteroids and sulphasalazine together with a suitable high protein and high calorie diet with additional supplements of vitamins and iron; others resort to surgery aimed at resecting the diseased area of the gut but endeavouring to preserve as much as possible. If the area adjacent to the caecum is involved then an ileo-rectal anastomosis may be possible, but if the rectum is affected then a proctocolectomy with permanent ileostomy may need to be undertaken; this latter may not need to be really permanent as the condition may improve with medical treatment for a year or so and

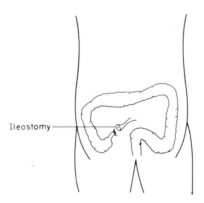

Fig. 56. *Ileostomy.*

provided a double-barrelled ileostomy has been raised this can be rejoined at a subsequent operation. Regional enteritis occurring in the large gut is likely to give rise to local complications, especially in the form of fistulae which may connect with coils of the small gut or form long tracks into the rectum or perineum. Also abscess formation is possible and these are usually peri-anal or ischio-rectal in position.

Fistula-in-ano

In this condition the track is lined with granulation tissue, and passes from deep in the anal canal or rectum to open superficially onto the skin around the anus; this is likely to be a high level fistula, one that is above the ano-rectal ring. Because the track is constantly becoming re-infected it fails to close. Prior to surgical treatment the gut must be prepared by the administration of antibiotics and washouts, and then at operation the track is opened along its length or as far as the ano-rectal ring (to incise this would lead to incontinence) and the lower edges packed with gauze. Skin grafts may be necessary around the anal wound. Some surgeons prefer not to insert an anal pack but to introduce a dilator daily following the first twenty-four hours after operation.

Peri-anal abscess

This is the result of infection in an anal gland which lies superficial to the external sphincter, and may originate from trauma or a blood

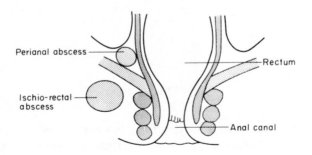

Fig. 57. *Position of perianal and ischiorectal abscesses.*

borne infection; it occurs in any age group. A cruciate incision over the abscess allows drainage to take place, and healing usually occurs in a few days.

Ischio-rectal abscess

This is the most painful of these three complications as the infection localizes in the ischio-rectal fossa which is mainly filled with fat; little distension of the tissues can occur. The abscess is palpated as a tender mass on the side of the anal canal and may give rise to generalized symptoms such as pyrexia. The abscess requires to be drained when the skin over the abscess is incised and the cavity explored. When the infection has subsided the area should be examined for the possibility of a fistula, in which case treatment should be given.

Nursing care

With all these conditions occurring in or around the anal canal it is important that the infected material be allowed to drain into a soft absorbent dressing which is changed frequently, and the actual track encouraged to granulate from the deeper towards the superficial tissues; if this does not happen the abscess is likely to recur. The patient may find difficulty in keeping a dressing in place but this is made easier with the use of Netelast cut to a pants shape or the use of a T-bandage. Whatever is used must be changed frequently as soiling is likely to occur. When drainage is completed, healing can be encouraged by the use of a bidet or sitting in the bath at least twice a day, and after each bowel action. A broad spectrum antibiotic will probably be prescribed, and the patient may need mild analgesia both before and immediately after the abscess has been incised. Care and attention to personal hygiene should be emphasized.

INTESTINAL PARASITES (Helminths)

A number of parasites use man as their host and choose some part of the alimentary tract in which to live and multiply. The most usual area is the intestine, both small and large, although some will be found in the liver. Many of these parasites also carry out part of their life cycle in animal tissues and it is mainly through ingestion of these or due to low standards of personal hygiene that man becomes infected. Adequate inspection and control over meat for human consumption followed by thorough cooking of all meat, plus the hygienic disposal of excreta and a high standard of personal cleanliness are measures which help to ensure that infection does not occur. Those parasites affecting the gastrointestinal tract will give rise to a number of different symptoms which are likely to include malabsorption, anaemia, weight loss and occasionally abdominal pain. In some instances the patient may be unaware that they have such a parasite, or they may be troubled by perianal irritation which prompts them to go to the doctor. Drugs used to rid the body of worms belong to the group known as the anthelmintics. The more common parasites occurring in the gastrointestinal tract of persons living in this country will be described in this chapter.

Tapeworm

There are two varieties, *Taenia saginata* which is found in beef, and *Taenia solium* in pork.

Taenia saginata
Man acquires the infection by ingesting larvae in infected meat. The larvae form cysts in the animal tissues and in these are found the future head of a new worm. The mature beef tapeworm may be up to 7 m (about 20 ft) in length, the head being attached by its four suction discs to the small intestinal mucosa. The body which is composed of many segments hangs freely along the lumen of the gut, segments containing many ova may break off and may be noted in the faeces and in this way a diagnosis is made. The presence of the worm (it is usually a single infection) causes vague gastrointestinal disturbance and anorexia, and in time will lead to general ill health and loss of weight.

Treatment. The aim of treatment must be to cause the head of the worm to be expelled, or it will simply renew the body segments within a period of three months. Drugs which may be used include:

Dichlorophen (Antiphen) 70 mg per kg body weight as a single dose, or in three divided doses over twenty-four hours.

Niclosamide (Yomesan) 1 g followed an hour later by a further 1 g . These two substances cause the worm to break up and the segments to be passed. The head is killed. Neither substance requires special preparation of the patient or the dose to be followed by a purge. Mepacrine hydrochloride and Male Fern may also be used but both require preparation in the form of a low residue diet, and the drug to be followed by a purge. Whichever form of treatment is used the stools must be carefully examined to note whether the head of the worm has been passed.

Taenia solium

This has a similar life cycle to that of *Taenia saginata* and is acquired by eating infected pork. This worm may have its larval stage (cysticercosis) in man, development taking place in the central nervous system, muscles and the eye. In all these areas serious damage can result. Dichlorophen and niclosamide are effective forms of treatment, but their use is discouraged due to their causing the worm to break up and thus liberating a large number of ova into the stools which may easily result in reinfection. Mepacrine hydrochloride or Male Fern should be used. The importance of a correct diagnosis being made before treatment to eradicate tapeworm is undertaken should be noted.

Hydatid cyst of liver

This is caused by the *Taenia echinococcus,* the adult form of which lives in the intestine of dogs and cats; segments of the worm are excreted in the animal's faeces and later become ingested by man. The embryo penetrates the wall of the small intestine, enters a blood vessel and is conveyed to the liver where cyst formation takes place. Cysts may also form in other organs such as the lungs, kidneys and stomach. Large cysts contain fluid and will give rise to a dragging pain in the abdomen due to their pressure; there is also local tissue damage and disturbance of function; in the liver this causes an increase in size which is painless. Diagnosis is made partly on the signs and symptoms, and specifically by the result of a complement fixation test or an intradermal reaction (Casoni test); a liver scan using radioactive gold will show a filling defect in the area of the cyst and aid diagnosis.

Treatment. The cyst is removed surgically having first aspirated the fluid, great care having been taken to prevent the spilling of fluid which could contaminate other tissues. There are no drugs suitable for the treatment of this condition.

Roundworm

Ascaris lumbricoides is a large white cylindrical worm about 25 cm in length which lives freely in the lumen of the intestine gaining its nutrition from the contents as they pass. Infection occurs by man ingesting the ova which may be present in dirt and dust. The ova hatch in the small intestine, the larvae may penetrate the intestinal wall, reach a blood vessel and be carried to the lungs. The larvae may be coughed up through the respiratory passages and are then swallowed, finally passing to the small intestine where they develop into adult worms. Presence of the worm may cause gastrointestinal discomfort and mild diarrhoea. Occasionally the worm enters the stomach and is vomited, or it may pass into the common bile duct causing obstruction and jaundice. Similarly it may obstruct the appendix. Diagnosis may be confirmed by finding ova in the patient's stools, or even an adult worm may be passed.

Treatment. Piperazine adipate 4 g orally as a single dose, followed by a purgative two hours later.

Dithiazanine iodide (Telmid) 50–100 mg orally four times a day for five days may also be used if treatment with piperazine has been unsuccessful.

Threadworm

Oxyuris vermicularis are very small worms measuring up to 10 mm in length and appear as slow moving white threads in the faeces, usually in large numbers. This is a condition which mainly occurs in children who ingest contaminated water and vegetables. The worms mature in the small intestine, and the female travels to the caecum and rectum, passing out of the anus to lay her fertilized eggs in the perianal region. As this mainly occurs at night and causes intense irritation this will lead to insomnia and irritability in the child. Re-infection frequently occurs as the child scratches and gets the ova under the finger nails and these may be put in the mouth.

Treatment. Piperazine adipate 0.5–1 g orally twice a day for seven days, or Pripsen 2–3 g orally as a single dose. Pripsen is a proprietary preparation of piperazine and contains Senokot which speeds the expulsion of the worms. Attention to hygiene is very important. The anal region should be washed thoroughly in the morning to remove any ova, and the child should wear cotton gloves at night to prevent scratching. Frequent laundering of the gloves and pyjamas is essential.

Hookworm

There are two main groups of hookworm, the *Ankylostoma duodenale* being more commonly found in people living in Europe. The worm is only 1 cm in length and is ingested in infected drinking water and uncooked vegetables; it is a condition associated with dirty living conditions and the presence of dried faeces. Larvae can enter through the skin and be conveyed in the blood vessels. The adult worm lives in the jejunum where it becomes mature within three to five weeks, and may pierce the mucosa causing bleeding. The patient may complain of gastrointestinal disturbances, accompanied by pain, fever, lethargy and anaemia.

Treatment. Tetrachloroethylene 1–3 ml orally as a single dose. This is followed two hours later by a saline aperient. As the treatment

H

may cause giddiness and drowsiness, the patient should be kept in bed. Food is withheld until the first stool has been passed.

Bephenium hydroxynaphthoate (Alcopar) 5 g orally in water as a single dose may also be given. The patient should have fasted overnight and no food given for two hours following the dose. An aperient is not required. With both these drugs treatment may not be successful on the first occasion and may need to be repeated.

Whipworm

The *Trichuris trichiura* is a common parasite of worldwide distribution. It is 5 cm in length and attaches itself to the intestinal wall by sinking its head deep into the mucosa and is usually to be found in the large intestine. Infection is acquired by swallowing ova about two weeks after they have been passed in human faeces. The embryos escape in the small intestine and pass on into the caecum and large intestine where if infection is severe they may cause diarrhoea, volvulus and sometimes rectal prolapse. Diagnosis is made by observing the presence of ova in the faeces.

Treatment. Dithiazanine iodide (Telmid) 50—100 mg orally four times a day for five days. This may cause nausea, diarrhoea and abdominal cramp, but is mainly non-toxic.

Trichiniasis

Trichinella spiralis. The larval stage of this worm is acquired by eating raw or underdone infected pork which contains cysts. The larvae are liberated into the duodenum and jejunum where they become attached to the mucosa. Adult worms are up to 3 mm in length, and the female bores through the intestinal mucosa to deposit embryos in the lacteals before she dies. The embryos are conveyed through the lymphatic vessels into the systemic circulation and become deposited in the tissues especially between the muscle fibres. The larvae develop inside cysts which cause muscle necrosis giving rise to pain and muscular weakness, often accompanied by pyrexia. The symptoms are at first gastrointestinal, the patient complains of nausea, colicky type pain and diarrhoea.

Treatment. In the early stages piperazine citrate 1—1·5 g orally twice daily for seven days. Steroids may also be given. The infection can be prevented by careful inspection of all pork flesh at the abattoir, and the adequate cooking of the pork.

NEOPLASTIC CONDITIONS

The incidence of tumours in the large intestine is high, the most common being the benign polyp and the malignant carcinoma.

Benign tumours

Polyps may be found in both the colon and rectum and occur mainly in the older age groups. Their distribution resembles that of carcinoma, and in fact the larger ones (over 3 cm in diameter) may become malignant in time. Polyps are chiefly of two types, those projecting from the mucosa—the papilloma, or the adenoma which is attached by a stalk to the underlying connective tissue. Both may cause symptoms of bleeding from the rectum, alteration in bowel habits and sometimes diarrhoea, although these features are more often found when carcinoma is present. Diagnosis is made during sigmoidoscopy if the polyp is situated in the distal part of the large intestine, or radiological examination (barium enema) may be necessary. All polyps should be removed, either by the use of the biopsy forceps at sigmoidoscopy or by performing a resection of the colon for those too high to be reached by this means. Radiological examination should always follow removal of polyps during sigmoidoscopy in order that additional ones or carcinoma are not ignored. Occasionally other benign tumours are present in the form of lipoma, fibroma and neurofibroma; these occur rarely but should always be removed if diagnosed.

Malignant tumours

A malignant tumour of the large intestine is one of the most commonly occurring malignant conditions and results in about 16 200 deaths each year. They occur mainly in the fifty-five to sixty age group, affecting men twice as frequently as women. Predisposing factors of their formation have been shown to be the presence of benign polyps, or familial polyposis of the colon (a hereditary condition occurring in the younger age group of between twenty and forty years and characterized by a large number of tumours present in the colon), and also as a complication of ulcerative colitis. Environmental factors have also been suggested as a possible cause, as well as certain toxic substances such as the long term use of liquid paraffin as an aperient.

These malignant tumours can be divided into four main groups according to their appearance.

(1) The nodular tumour which juts out into the lumen of the gut. Its surface is likely to become ulcerated, bleed and become infected producing pus. The tumour may grow into a large ulcerated mass with a necrotic base.

(2) The colloid tumour which undergoes mucoid degeneration and becomes gelatinous in appearance.

(3) the scirrhus tumour in which a fibrous reaction has taken place; this tumour commonly encircles the gut.

(4) The polypoid tumour which is attached by its pedicle to the gut wall has probably developed from an existing polyp.

Malignant tumours are more likely to occur in the rectum and pelvic or sigmoid colon than in the transverse and ascending colon, and all are capable of producing metastases either as a result of direct invasion of the tissues or spread by the blood or lymphatic channels, this latter being the most common. These malignant tumours may also be graded according to the extent of their development:

Grade I—the tumour is confined to the bowel wall and has not formed metastases.

Grade II—the tumour has penetrated the bowel wall but still has not produced metastases.

Grade III—metastases are present in the regional lymph nodes.

Grade IV—distant metastases have been formed; these are often present in the liver.

The symptoms produced by the tumours vary according to the part of the colon in which they are to be found. The ascending colon has a large lumen and therefore obstruction is unlikely to occur with a tumour situated here, but the patient may complain of abdominal pain, weight loss, a general feeling of malaise probably accompanied by pyrexia, and also be found to have anaemia. Tumours in the descending colon which is considerably narrower in its lumen, are more likely to cause a degree of obstruction which results in pain, and alteration in bowel habits accompanied by either diarrhoea or constipation or alternating between the two. Malignant tumours in the rectum will probably cause bleeding as well as an alteration in bowel habits, but obstruction is less likely to occur and pain is an unusual feature.

Diagnosis

Diagnosis of tumours in the large intestine can be made by palpating a large mass in the abdomen, digital examination of the rectum, sigmoidoscopy, and a barium enema which shows a filling defect. To these investigations can be added colonoscopy in which the colon is viewed through a flexible fibre-optic colonoscope (see page 287), examination of cells acquired during colonic lavage, and the presence of occult blood in the stools. Ascites may also be present. It must be remembered that the conditions of ulcerative colitis and haemorrhoids may also give positive results to some of these tests and it is important that a correct differential diagnosis is made.

Treatment

The choice of treatment depends on the site of the carcinoma, the stage of its development and the age and general condition of the patient. The methods of treatment are mainly surgical removal of the tumour, or if this is impossible then radiotherapy may be given to reduce the size of the growth and discourage its invasive tendencies. If the tumour is in the early non-invasive stage then a resection of the colon and anastomosis is carried out, the growth being removed and the lymph nodes excised as far back as the aorta. The prognosis is better if this type of treatment can be given, about two-thirds of the patients so treated being alive and well five years later. Unfortunately for many, diagnosis is not made until the tumour is well advanced in which case the operation of choice may need to be an abdomino-perineal excision of rectum with the formation of a permanent colostomy. The patients for whom extensive surgery is contra-indicated will probably be treated by radiotherapy and the raising of a colostomy to overcome obstruction in the lower bowel.

Less common malignant tumours

Other tumours which may occur in the bowel are the squamous cell carcinoma which is usually to be found in the anal canal where it causes painful defaecation and bleeding, a sarcoma, and finally an argentaffinoma; this latter may be present in either the colon or rectum and the methods of treatment resemble those for carcinoma.

Nursing care

Surgery of the large bowel is usually extensive being carried out on patients who are far from being fit, and added to this is their fear and worry associated with not only the idea of having, but also caring for a colostomy. The nurse will need to be extremely patient in her approach to the sick person, and be prepared to repeat time and again what the operation and subsequent care involves. When a diagnosis has been made following a full range of investigations available, then preparation for surgery can begin. Mainly this involves improving the patient's general condition by correcting anaemia and giving a high calorie diet to replace some of the lost weight and observing that an adequate amount of fluid is taken each day. Local preparation of the bowel is accomplished by giving a low residue diet, a daily enema or washout, and the use of drugs such as phthalylsulphathiazole up to 2 g orally every four or six hours, or neomycin $\frac{1}{2}-1$ mega unit orally, four hourly to prepare the gut. During this preparatory period a chest X-ray should be taken, and an intravenous pyelogram carried out to exclude involvement of the ureters by the tumour. A sample of blood should be taken for haemoglobin estimation, and blood cross-matched ready for transfusion during and after the operation. Immediately prior to going to theatre the abdomen and perineal area should be shaved, a Ryle's tube passed into the stomach and left spigotted, and an indwelling catheter (usually a Foley catheter) passed into the bladder. The patient is then prepared in the usual way for theatre.

Following operation the patient will return to the ward with possibly three wounds; these are the abdominal incision which may or may not have a drainage tube close by, the colostomy, usually covered by a transparent plastic bag attached to the surrounding skin and through which the stoma is readily observed; and finally the perineal wound which may contain a drainage tube or gauze pack. When consciousness has been regained the patient is nursed preferably in the semi-recumbent position, inclined to one side, so that regular turning to the other buttock can take place and the body weight is therefore not taken directly by the perineum. The patient may find it comfortable to sit on a foam ring. In the immediate postoperative period the stomach contents will be aspirated at intervals, and only when bowel sounds return should small quantities of fluid be offered by mouth. During this time the intravenous infusion will have been continued until a satisfactory fluid intake by mouth allows the patient to have the Ryle's tube removed and to be offered a light, then normal diet. Care of the indwelling catheter will need to be given in an aseptic manner at least twice a day, and provided the patient is making satisfactory progress the catheter may be removed on about the fifth post-operative day, after which careful note must be made of the ability to pass urine normally. Broad spectrum antibiotics will be given to prevent infection occurring in either the respiratory or renal tracts or the operative area. Analgesia will be needed as the patient is likely to experience considerable discomfort at first from the wounds and drainage devices, and suitable narcotics should be given, changing to less strong analgesia as soon as the patient has less severe pain. Mobilization may be difficult in the early stages but movements should be encouraged and the physiotherapist will play an important role in the post-operative care of this patient.

The care of the abdominal wound and the drainage tube will follow a normal pattern; the colostomy will probably not work for about forty-eight hours and then be rather erratic in its timing and amount excreted; this should improve when the patient becomes established once again on a normal diet, but the area which will take longest to heal is the perineal wound. It is important that granulation occurs from the apex, and so following removal of the drainage tube or pack the wound may be irrigated twice daily using a solution such as hypochlorite which helps to clean the sinus as well as promote healing. Once the patient is mobile he can be assisted to take a bath which will be beneficial to the perineal wound. It must be appreciated that the patient is likely to feel depressed during the early post-operative period; the discomfort of the sore perineum and the apparent slow rate of healing, together with the irregularity of action of the colostomy appear as never ending problems. The nurse will need to give much support and encouragement, but not be too enthusiastic to get a frail, elderly person to care for their colostomy; this will come in time when the patient has had opportunity to really adjust to the new situation. The patient will benefit from an unhurried post-operative period followed by convalescence if this can be arranged. For detailed care of the colostomy the reader is referred to Chapter 10.

HAEMORRHOIDS

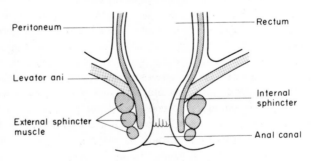

Fig. 58. *Anal canal.*

Haemorrhoids or piles, are varicose veins which occur in the plexuses of veins draining the anal canal and lower rectum. They may be divided into two main groups, internal and external.

Internal haemorrhoids

These occur in dilatations of the lower tributaries of the superior haemorrhoidal vein of the internal haemorrhoidal plexus. There are three main positions for haemorrhoids occurring here which correspond to the position of the main veins. These have often been described as occurring at 3, 7 and 11 o'clock, but secondary haemorrhoids may occupy the intervening spaces. Haemorrhoids do occur in young people, but by far the majority occur in the

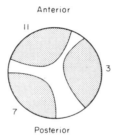

Fig. 59. *Position of haemorrhoids.*

middle and latter years of life, a number of factors predisposing to their formation:

(1) Hereditary. There is often a family history of this condition.

(2) Chronic constipation resulting in straining to defaecate. Similarly straining to micturate in cases of chronic prostatic obstruction.

(3) The presence of pelvic tumours, especially a pregnancy, where the venous return has a considerable obstacle to negotiate.

(4) Continual rise in intra-abdominal pressure as is noted in men doing heavy manual work.

(5) In portal hypertension where the vessels forming the internal haemorrhoidal plexus undergo dilatation in order to function as collateral vessels and thus help to relieve the situation.

(6) Carcinoma of the rectum may be associated with the formation of haemorrhoids; this factor must never be overlooked when making a diagnosis of the latter.

Internal haemorrhoids may be classified according to the extent of prolapse which occurs:

First degree haemorrhoids do not prolapse through the anal sphincter, their main symptom being that of bleeding which occurs as a bright red loss at the time of defaecation. If this situation continues for several months it may lead to iron deficiency anaemia.

Second degree haemorrhoids prolapse during defaecation and either return spontaneously or are easily replaced. Pain is present during the temporary prolapse but not at other times.

Third degree haemorrhoids are permanently prolapsed, and in these the covering mucosa often becomes thicker and secretes more mucus which causes pruritus. The prolapsed haemorrhoid may undergo venous thrombosis appearing as a large purple mass which is very painful; this is often referred to as a strangulated pile or by the patient as 'having an attack of piles', thrombosis having occurred because the base of the haemorrhoid has become nipped by the anal sphincter. Diagnosis is made partly by the history given by the patient, and also during examination through a proctoscope.

Treatment of haemorrhoids may be either by local injection or surgery. Injection is really only suitable for first degree haemorrhoids, and is a painless form of treatment although some discomfort will probably be experienced. The rectum should be empty but no other preparation is necessary. An injection of 3–5 ml 5% phenol in almond oil is given into the submucous tissue above the level of the haemorrhoid, and not into the haemorrhoid itself. A little bleeding from the injection site is likely but no further local treatment is indicated, only that of the predisposing factors if this is relevant.

Surgical treatment for haemorrhoids involves their removal, the operation of haemorrhoidectomy. The patient is usually admitted two days before operation so that preparation can be undertaken.

The patient is given an aperient on the evening of admission, followed by an enema during the day prior to surgery, and then a rectal washout as part of the immediate preparation for theatre. The perineal area should be shaved. The patient's haemoglobin level should also be estimated. During the operation the anal sphincter is dilated, the haemorrhoids ligated and removed, the stumps being returned to the anal canal. This operation leaves a bare skin area from where each haemorrhoid has been excised which may take up to six weeks to heal completely. After the operation pieces of vaseline gauze are tucked into the anus by one corner and arranged in a radiating fashion over the raw areas, a gauze and wool pad is applied on top and the whole kept in place with Netelast or a T-bandage.

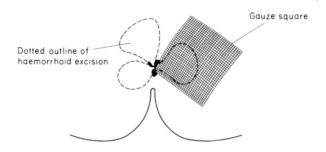

Fig. 60. *Arrangement of haemorrhoidectomy dressing.*

Nursing care

The patient may complain of severe pain at first on regaining consciousness and may require an analgesic such as pethidine hydrochloride, but as time passes less strong analgesia will be found to be sufficient. Reactionary haemorrhage is more likely to occur than a secondary haemorrhage for this patient, and therefore the nurse should make frequent observations on the anal dressing and pad as well as recording the rate and volume of the pulse during the first few hours after return to the ward. If haemorrhage does occur, it may be controlled by an intravenous injection of morphine sulphate; if not the patient will need to return to theatre so that the bleeding vessels can be located and ligated. Retention of urine may occur at first after operation; this is more likely in the male patient and may be relieved by giving carbachol if other usual nursing methods fail. The patient will be assisted to have a bath during the day following operation, when the dressings will be encouraged to soak off, and then be replaced by dry dressings in the same manner as previously. Baths and redressing of the area continue twice a day and after every bowel action, until the patient is discharged from hospital on about the tenth or twelfth day. A mild aperient such as liquid paraffin is started on the second post-operative evening and continued each day until just before discharge home. This should enable a soft stool to be passed with the minimum of discomfort, and although constipation should be avoided the patient should be encouraged to pass a more formed stool without the continual use of aperients. A week after operation a digital examination is carried out to assess the degree of anal spasm and the possibility of stricture formation. The anus is dilated with a St Mark's Hospital dilator and

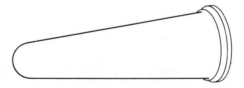

Fig. 61. *St Mark's anal dilator.*

the patient is instructed how to carry this out for himself. On discharge from hospital the patient should be advised to take a daily bath, be able to use the anal dilator correctly, and know how to reapply a gauze dressing, having been given an adequate supply of these. An appointment should be made to see him in the outpatient department one month later, when he should be fit and well, not requiring further use of the anal dilator and possibly only needing a small gauze dressing.

External haemorrhoids

The acute external haemorrhoid or perianal haematoma is caused by rupture of the inferior haemorrhoidal vein into the subcutaneous tissues of the anal canal; this usually occurs during straining to defaecate. The haematoma form a tense, bluish swelling which is very painful and if it becomes infected will form a perianal abscess. The haematoma may resolve spontaneously in a few days, or possibly the overlying skin may necrose and allow the clot to be extruded; if this does not happen then a local anaesthetic may be given before an incision and evacuation of the haematoma is carried out. Following this the patient is advised to take twice daily baths and apply a clean gauze dressing to the area. Attention to the underlying constipation will also be necessary.

Rectal prolapse

This condition is likely to result from continual straining to defaecate, or in cases of chronic diarrhoea. It may also occur in the elderly where there is loss of anal tone, and in those suffering from severe malnutrition. In partial rectal prolapse only the rectal mucosa and submucosa project through the anus for a distance of about 2·5 cm. Treatment is mainly to remedy the cause of the abnormal bowel action, and if possible encourage excercises to strengthen the muscles of the pelvic floor. In complete rectal prolapse the entire thickness of the rectal wall prolapses to a distance of 7·5 cm or more. This also occurs in debilitating diseases and also in women with extensive pelvic floor injury following traumatic childbirth. Following reduction of the prolapse, the treatment as for partial prolapse may be sufficient; if not surgery to effect an adequate repair will be necessary.

Anal fissure

The term describes a narrow triangular ulcer present in the anal mucosa, the apex at the lower border of the internal sphincter and the base situated at the anal margin. Often there is an area of swollen mucosa projecting as a skin tag through the anus from alongside it; this is known as a sentinel pile. Anal fissure usually occurs in the middle-aged who suffer from chronic constipation, and severe pain is experienced during defaecation. The constipation often becomes worse as the act of defaecation is delayed in order not to experience the severe pain which always accompanies it. Examination of the anus should only be made after the application of a local anaesthetic such as 5% xylocaine jelly, even so it it too painful to use a proctoscope.

Treatment consists of dilating the anal sphincter to allow the fissure to close and not re-open with each bowel movement. Dilatation can be carried out twice daily by the patient having been shown how to insert the St Mark's Hospital dilator after applying the anaesthetic gel. This treatment should be continued for a month, by which time the fissure should be healed. Suitable aperients should also be taken to encourage the formation of a soft stool which is easily passed. If for some reason this treatment is unsuitable for the patient then dilatation will be carried out under general anaesthesia; this may be all that is required or the surgeon may need to divide the muscle fibres in the floor of the fissure and remove the sentinel pile. Following operation the patient will need to have the anus dilated each day and take a daily bath, and also take suitable aperients to enable a comfortable bowel action. Healing usually takes place within three weeks.

CHAPTER 10

Stoma Care

An ever-increasing number of persons both young and old are finding that they are having to adjust to life with a stoma, and many nurses now realize that they have a special role with regard to the care and psychological support that these patients need. The stoma may be that of an ileostomy, colostomy or urinary diversion, surgery having been undertaken for treatment of inflammatory disease or carcinoma of the bowel, or a malignant tumour of the bladder. In recent years improved methods of diagnosis have meant that more patients with ulcerative colitis or Crohn's disease have been able to receive treatment, but the stress of everyday living has contributed to the psychological problems that many of these patients have experienced. In the very early stages of life, babies with neurological disorders such as spina bifida and meningocele are surviving but may require surgery in the form of a urinary diversion in order to make their life more tolerable.

The nurse who has the charge of stoma patients has a responsibility for their nursing care in the immediate pre- and post-operative period, to help them adjust to the new situation by appreciating their psychological and psychiatric problems, as well as giving the necessary help and advice over any social difficulties; and by no means least of all the nurse must help in the rehabilitation of her patients and encourage them to continue as active members of the community. These functions of the nurse mean that she needs to acquire expertise in stoma care and be able to pass on this technical skill to the patient and his family. Because of the growing awareness of this particular field of nursing, special training courses are available. The successful rehabilitation of a stoma patient must be regarded as a team effort between all members of the medical and nursing staff involved in the total care of the patient.

The colostomy

This may be either permanent or temporary.

Permanent colostomy

The formation of this type of colostomy is usually part of an extensive operation for carcinoma of the rectum, when an abdomino-perineal excision of the rectum is performed. The stoma is situated in the left iliac fossa and the rectum is removed.

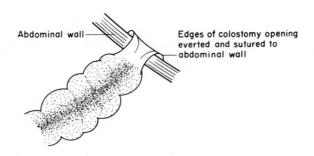

Fig. 62. *Terminal (permanent) colostomy.*

Temporary colostomy

This may be performed to allow the bowel to rest in situations of inflammatory disease or where an anastomosis needs time to heal. Sometimes it is used to relieve an obstruction. The transverse colon is brought onto the surface of the abdomen usually just below the umbilicus and to the right of the midline, the loop of bowel being supported on a glass rod. The colon is then incised and the mucosa sutured to the skin. This type of colostomy allows for closure at a later date and a return to normal bowel function.

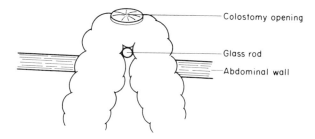

Fig. 63. *Loop (temporary) colostomy.*

The ileostomy

This too may be either permanent or temporary.

Permanent ileostomy

In this instance the whole of the large intestine is removed, an operation carried out for severe ulcerative colitis or Crohn's disease. The stoma is sited just below the level of the umbilicus and to the right of the midline.

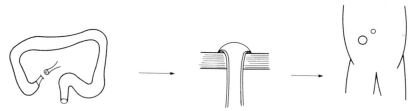

Fig. 64. *Permanent ileostomy.*

Temporary ileostomy

As with the temporary colostomy this is usually performed to allow a period of rest in which an anastomosis of the gut is able to heal. It too is held in place with a glass rod and may be a little closer to the midline than the permanent type.

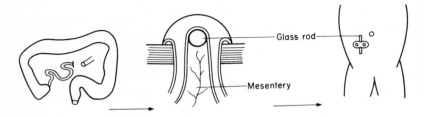

Fig. 65. *Temporary ileostomy.*

The ileal conduit
The stoma that results from urinary diversion is usually formed from part of the ileum which has been isolated from the remainder of the small intestine to form a reservoir for urine following transplantation of the ureters from the bladder into this loop of gut.

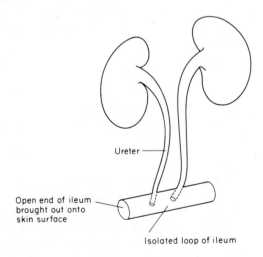

Fig. 66. *Ileal conduit.*

Pre-stoma preparation

Pre-operatively the most ideal site for the stoma must be agreed bearing in mind that the appliance must fit closely all round so that leakage is avoided, and that it does not form a bulge under clothing. The surgeon should avoid the costal margin, siting the stoma too close to the umbilicus, over the iliac crests or in the vicinity of previous scars; all of these will prevent the appliance fitting snugly to the abdominal wall. The ideal site is just below the belt line and a little to one side of the midline. Some surgeons prefer the patient to be shown the appliances and to wear one for a period of time whilst normal movements are carried on so that the most suitable site is found. It is vitally important that the stoma is situated correctly, for any leakage from the appliance will cause skin excoriation to occur and may produce untold discomfort and misery for the patient; with care in the pre-operative period all of this can be avoided. Besides determining the site of the stoma the patient needs to be prepared psychologically. The nurse can help by answering questions promptly and correctly (and maybe repeat this information several times) so that the patient can voice his fears and anxieties and come to terms with the idea of an abdominal stoma. It may be suitable for the patient to be visited by someone who finds no difficulty in coping with their stoma and who has a sensible approach to the situation. The nurse will be required to assess her patient's needs in this respect, and what is suitable for one may not be so for another, and even more anxiety may be created by the wrong approach. The relatives must also be included in this preparatory period, for they too will have queries to be answered, and in many cases when suitably informed will be able to give added support to the patient.

Post-stoma care

Whilst the patient is in theatre a transparent drainage bag will be fitted, and this should be the type that can be emptied without removal as it may stay in place for up to one week initially. The discharge will be fluid at first and the bag will require emptying at regular intervals, the contents being measured and recorded. The transparent bag will allow for ease of observation of the stoma which will probably be oedematous at first but after a few days should become a healthy pink colour. Any discolouration of the stoma should be reported immediately as this indicates an inadequate blood supply. The colostomy and ileostomy will not begin to act until peristalsis returns, and as the discharge is fluid at first it is important to see that the patient does not become dehydrated. After a time the discharge from the permanent colostomy becomes formed and there may be one or two stools a day, but that from the temporary colostomy (transverse colon) may only be semiformed and therefore needs to be managed in the same way as an ileostomy. The ileostomy discharge will be copious and fluid at first, becoming semiformed later. From an ileal conduit urine is excreted continuously. Sometimes infection occurs around the stoma in the early stages, but this usually clears within a few weeks.

Diet. The patient should be encouraged to eat normally, having well balanced meals. Extra fluid should be taken to compensate for that lost in the semiformed stools. Certain foods should be eaten in moderation or avoided, especially onions, fish, brussel sprouts and cabbage; for many patients these cause flatus, diarrhoea and unpleasant odour. If diarrhoea occurs then extra fluid and salt should be taken, and a doctor consulted if the situation has not resolved within forty-eight hours. Isogel or methylcellulose (Celevac) may be prescribed for occasional use if the stools are fluid; these are bulk substances and act by absorbing water and therefore help solidify the stool.

Selecting the appliance
When choosing the appliance three things must be taken into account:
   (1) It must be leakproof;
   (2) It must not be obvious under clothing and cause embarrassment;
   (3) It must be easy for the patient to deal with.
The patient should be allowed to select what suits him from the range of appliances available, and he is likely to choose one that is

light in weight, easy to handle, comfortable and safe to wear. The choice also depends on the type of stoma, but the patient must remember that if the flange is too small it may damage the stoma and if too large leakage will occur and cause excoriation of the surrounding skin; ideally the flange should be 0·625 cm (quarter inch) larger in diameter than the stoma.

Colostomy appliances. When the stools have become formed the patient may prefer to simply wear a dry dressing, as with a well regulated colostomy the patient can deal with it at a suitable time each day; otherwise an appliance may be worn, the bag being either self adhesive or attached to a ring and belt.

Ileostomy and ileal conduit appliances. These must be leakproof, and ideally consist of a rubber bag with a stopper for ease of emptying.

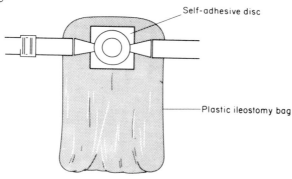

Fig. 67. *Ileostomy appliance (self-adhesive).*

Changing the appliance. Whatever type of appliance is used the area of skin around the stoma must be thoroughly washed with soap and water and then dried carefully. No ether or spirit should be used for cleaning the skin. When a disposable bag is used it should be carefully peeled off the skin starting from above, the bag is then cut across at the top to allow easy disposal of the contents into the toilet, the bag is then well wrapped in paper and either incinerated or placed in the dustbin. For the non-disposable type of appliance the

new bag should be assembled first. The flange should be cleaned
with methylated ether to remove traces of adhesive and all conta-
minants. A hole is cut in the stomaseal to the same size as the flange,
then the backing is removed and the stomaseal applied to the flange.

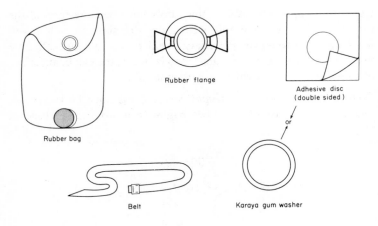

Fig. 68. *Ileostomy appliances.*

The used appliance is now removed in one piece and the skin
washed and dried. A Karaya gum disc may be placed around the
stoma to protect the skin. The protective paper can now be removed
from the stomaseal and the appliance centred over the stoma and
pressed into position, care being taken to avoid creasing or conta-
minating it. Micropore, or other adhesive may be used to give
reinforcement, and finally a belt may be worn to provide extra
support. The used bag should be rinsed under running water then
turned inside out and washed in warm soapy water and then dried
thoroughly and powdered to prevent perishing. Changing the whole
appliance should not be necessary more than twice a week and
possibly less often. As soon as possible after operation the patient

should be encouraged to empty the bag as this gives him a certain degree of independence. The patient must be encouraged to take an interest in the changing of the bag, and the nurses' attitude when doing this in the initial stages is very important as this may leave a lasting impression on the patient. As soon as the patient is physically fit and psychologically ready he should be encouraged to take over the care of the stoma. Each stage will need careful demonstration and maybe repeating several times until he feels confident to take over. It is often a good idea to have a relative there as well so that they receive the same tuition and can give advice and encouragement when the patient returns home. Whilst teaching the patient care of the stoma the nurse has an excellent opportunity to encourage a high standard of personal hygiene and to impress the need for the correct disposal of used equipment. The patient will certainly need access to the bathroom when at home and will probably find it easier to keep all the necessary equipment together on a tray.

Renewal of equipment. When the patient leaves hospital he should be given an ample supply of appliances (usually sufficient for one month) and also a list of everything he needs. He should know that further supplies are available on a prescription obtained from his doctor, and for which no financial charge is made. The general practitioner should be notified of the patient's diagnosis, treatment and after care required, and also the home nurse will be asked to visit if it is thought necessary.

Advising the patient. Many patients find security in belonging to an organization composed of people with a similar problem, and two voluntary organizations exist for this purpose namely, the Ileostomy Association founded in the early 1950s and the Colostomy Welfare Group started in 1965. Both of these bodies give a lot of psychological support to new stoma patients and some very real practical advice concerning how to deal with problems that may arise, and also distribute information about new and improved appliances as they become available. In some hospitals a stoma clinic is held to which patients are encouraged to come and obtain advice from the stomatherapist.

Colostomy washout

Occasionally it may be necessary to carry out a washout either to encourage an action in a recently established colostomy or to relieve constipation. The patient should sit comfortably with a kidney dish supported under the stoma and a bucket close at hand. Warm water or normal saline is allowed to run through to the end of a catheter (size 20FG, 12EG) attached to a funnel, tubing and connection and then the catheter is gently introduced into the stoma for a distance of approximately 15 cm. About 500 ml of fluid is run in gently, the catheter removed and the fluid with faecal content allowed to run out into the dish. When all has been returned, the surrounding skin is cleaned and dried and the usual protection applied.

Problems. It is almost inevitable that at some time problems will arise for which the patient will seek professional advice. These may include:

(1) The stoma has slipped back and does not extend the normal 2–3 cm from the surface of the abdomen, and because of this fluid leaks under the appliance. Surgery may be needed to correct this.

(2) The stoma prolapses and therefore makes for difficulty in fitting the appliance which also may cause damage to the stoma. This may need surgical correction.

(3) Leakage onto the skin causing excoriation. With a well fitting appliance and care in handling this should not happen, but when it does occur the skin can be protected with a barrier cream, Karaya gum powder, Friar's Balsam, calamine lotion or a protective adhesive square in which a hole has been cut.

(4) Erythema may occur as a result of contact dermatitis. This patient should be seen by the dermatologist in order that the cause can be identified and removed. If the surrounding skin area has become infected then application of an antibiotic cream may be necessary.

CHAPTER 11

Hernia

Hernia is the term used to describe the protrusion of an organ or part of an organ through an abnormal opening. A hernia may occur in a number of places in the body such as the brain, bladder or through an incision, but in this chapter only the common herniations of parts of the gastrointestinal tract will be considered. The structures which herniate mainly consist of three items—the actual gut, the gut contents and the tissue covering the whole which is usually peritoneum.

Hernia may be of several types:

Reducible hernia

When the patient lies down the hernia reduces itself but will recur when the patient stands. Sometimes the hernia does not do this for itself but can be easily replaced by the patient.

Irreducible hernia

In this case the contents of the hernia cannot be replaced. Attempts to reduce the hernia result only in partial replacement which in some instances could lead to strangulation. It is more usual in a femoral or umbilical hernia.

Obstructed hernia

The contents of the loop of bowel which herniates are arrested in their passage along the gut and thus cause intestinal obstruction. At first there is no interference with the blood supply to the gut wall, but the condition may progress to that of strangulation.

Strangulated hernia

Here, the blood supply to the gut wall is seriously impaired so that gangrene of the bowel is a possible outcome. At first the venous return is impaired, therefore the wall becomes congested and bright red in colour, and serous fluid is poured into the hernial sac. As the condition progresses the loop of gut becomes more distended and the wall a purple colour and is further aggravated by a reduced arterial supply to the intestinal wall and blood effusing into the serous fluid in the sac and into the lumen of the loop. Because of the tension the gut wall becomes atonic and friable, and bacteria migrate into the fluid. Gangrene may commence at the point of maximum constriction of the gut, and as decomposition of the blood in that area takes place so the characteristic colour change to greenish–black occurs. If the situation is unrelieved perforation of the wall may occur, liberating the contents into the peritoneal cavity and predisposing to peritonitis.

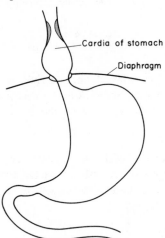

Fig. 69. *'Sliding' hernia.*

Hiatus hernia

Hiatus hernia is a situation where part of the stomach herniates through the oesophageal opening in the diaphragm, and in doing so allows reflux of gastric acid into the oesophagus causing ulceration. There are two types of hiatus hernia:

Hiatal hernia (sliding) in which part of the stomach protrudes through the diaphragm and lies alongside the oesophagus.

Para-oesophageal hernia (rolling) in which the stomach herniates

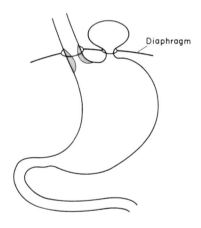

Diaphragm

Fig. 70. *'Rolling' hernia.*

through a second opening in the diaphragm close to the oesophageal one.

Eventration is a condition in which the stomach bulges under the diaphragm but does not actually herniate through it.

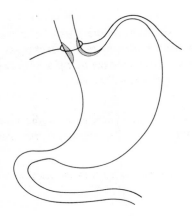

Fig. 71. *Eventration.*

Hiatus hernia occurs as a congenital abnormality in about one in one thousand babies, whereas forty per cent of adults have this condition. The reflux of gastric acid causes oesophagitis which gives rise to retrosternal burning pain, pain on lying flat or bending down (postural pain) and pain on swallowing hot liquids or alcohol. Diagnosis of the condition is made by taking a careful history of the symptoms, a barium swallow to demonstrate the reflux into the oesophagus when the head is tilted downwards, and an oesophagos-copy when the oesophagitis can be viewed and a biopsy taken.

Treatment. The patient should be encouraged to adopt an upright posture and become used to bending from the knees instead of stooping, and should also sleep with several pillows. Antacids should be taken when necessary, at hourly intervals if need be. It is preferable to give a mixture of magnesium and calcium salts as individually they are likely to give rise to symptoms of diarrhoea, constipation or alkalosis. Many patients are obese, and reduction of weight should be encouraged along with the taking of smaller, more frequent meals.

Surgery may need to be undertaken to correct the condition if medical methods fail. Besides returning the stomach into the abdominal cavity the surgeon needs to refashion the angle between the oesophagus and the fundus of the stomach, and repair the hiatus. Oesophageal stricture sometimes complicates the condition and may be treated by dilatation or resection of the affected area and anastomosis to the stomach.

Hiatus hernia in babies (partial thoracic stomach)
Occasionally a hiatus hernia occurs in infants and will be diagnosed soon after birth. It affects babies of either sex and occurs about one in one thousand births; it may be associated with other congenital anomalies or prematurity. The baby usually takes its feeds well but effortless vomiting occurs when the baby is laid flat in the cot; the vomit may be specked with blood. The amount of vomit may be small and not detrimental to the baby's health, but if the vomiting is copious or the situation is allowed to continue then hunger and failure to thrive will be apparent. Surgical treatment is not indicated at this stage as invariably as the baby gets bigger the condition improves. In the meantime the baby should sleep in a reclining

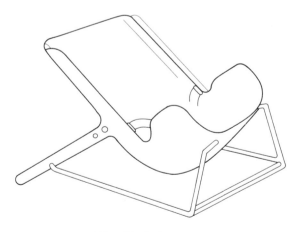

Fig. 72. *Baby 'sitta'.*

position (at an angle of sixty degrees) being suitably supported by firm pillows, or be placed in a 'Baby Sitta' in the cot, care being taken to see that he is strapped in. This treatment should be continued until the baby has been symptom-free for six weeks. The mother may be concerned that the baby will suffer postural damage by being allowed to sit up at such an early age. She should be encouraged to lay the baby on a flat surface at any time other than immediately after a feed. If the baby continues to vomit then the feeds should be thickened slightly or early weaning commenced, so that less fluid need be given at each feed. If the condition has not corrected itself by the time the baby is twelve months old then surgery may be indicated, the operation aiming to prevent gastro-oesophageal reflux or relieve an oesophageal stricture if this has formed.

Inguinal hernia

The inguinal canal

This is an oblique passage through the muscle layers of the lower abdominal wall through which the spermatic cord passes in the male and the round ligament in the female, accompanied in both cases by the ilio-inguinal nerve. The canal is 3·75 cm in length and extends

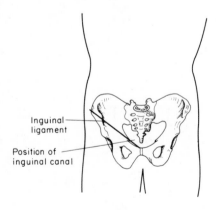

Inguinal ligament

Position of inguinal canal

Fig. 73. *Position of inguinal canal.*

between two openings, the internal and external inguinal rings, lying parallel to and immediately above the inguinal ligament which joins the anterior superior spine to the pubic tubercle.

The abdominal wall is formed of several layers; in front of the canal are the skin and superficial tissues overlying the external oblique aponeurosis together with the internal oblique muscle covering the lateral one-third of the canal, whilst behind and above are the transversalis fascia and the transversus muscle (this latter joins the internal oblique muscle).

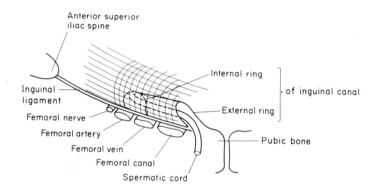

Fig. 74. *Right inguinal canal.*

The canal is bounded by two 'rings', the internal ring which lies midway between the symphysis pubis and the anterior superior iliac spine and is the point at which the spermatic cord or round ligament push their way through the transversalis fascia; and the external ring which is a V-shaped opening in the external oblique aponeurosis immediately above the pubic tubercle.

Types of inguinal hernia

Indirect

This is the most common of all herniae, occurring twenty times more frequently in men than in women. In about one third of cases it is bilateral, and occurs in infants as well as adults. The loop of gut passes through the internal ring and along the inguinal canal, finally emerging at the external ring; in the male it may pass on into the scrotum. If the hernia can be reduced, it may be controlled by finger-tip pressure over the internal ring. (This may be located immediately above the point where the femoral artery passes under the inguinal ligament, pressure being applied about 1 cm above the femoral pulse.)

Direct

The loop of gut is pushed directly forwards from behind the inguinal canal, and if the hernia is large enough it will push through the external ring into the scrotum. Only about one-tenth of inguinal herniae are of the direct type and are acquired by adults, predisposing factors being chronic cough, straining and heavy manual work. This type of hernia is very rare in women.

Clinical features of inguinal hernia

Pain may be felt in the groin or testis during strenuous exercise or whilst doing heavy manual work, and a small bulge may be seen over the inguinal region when the patient coughs. Later, the hernia may protrude as soon as the patient stands upright and this may be accompanied by a feeling of weight and epigastric pain. In babies the hernia appears as a swelling when the baby cries.

Treatment of inguinal hernia

Indirect hernia

Truss. This may be used when operation is contraindicated for some reason such as age or general condition. The hernia must be able to be reduced as the truss exerts pressure over the inguinal canal thus preventing protrusion of the gut through it. The patient must be instructed to put the truss on before getting up in the morning and to wear it all day, it is also important that it fits correctly and is kept in a satisfactory state of repair. If the truss does not fit well then it may cause strangulation of the hernia.

Surgical treatment. Herniotomy entails opening out the hernial sac, reducing any contents present, tying off the neck of the sac to retain the gut in the abdomen and then removing any excess sac. This operation is suitable for infants and young adults where there is good muscle tone of the abdominal wall, but is used as preliminary to herniorrhaphy for adults. In babies the internal and external inguinal rings are superimposed and therefore it is unnecessary to open the inguinal canal.

Herniorrhaphy and hernioplasty really consist of three operations, first a herniotomy, then the repair of the transversalis fascia to reduce the size of the internal inguinal ring, followed by reconstruction of the posterior wall of the inguinal canal. The hernioplasty may be carried out by using sutures, a flap of fascia, stainless steel wire or Dacron net.

Direct hernia

Surgical techniques are similar to those employed for indirect hernia except that the hernial sac is not removed, it is simply replaced in the abdomen and the transversalis fascia repaired over it. It is necessary to reconstruct the posterior wall of the inguinal canal.

Strangulated inguinal hernia

This may occur at any age and in either sex. It is usually caused by a loop of small intestine herniating as the indirect variety. This is an emergency and requires urgent operation, although if the patient is grossly dehydrated the surgeon may prefer to wait two or three hours whilst resuscitative measures are undertaken; these include correction of dehydration and electrolyte imbalance by the administration of intravenous fluids, and gastric aspiration. The bladder should be emptied and catheterization may be necessary. At operation the constriction is relieved and the intestine inspected for viability, if this is satisfactory the loop of gut is returned to the abdomen and a herniorrhaphy performed to close the hernial sac. A

I

gangrenous length of gut will need to be resected and an anasto-mosis carried out prior to replacing it in the abdominal cavity.

Femoral hernia

Femoral hernia accounts for about 20% of all herniae occurring in women, but for only 5% in men, it occurs chiefly on the right side although 20% are bilateral. The female pelvis is wider than the male, therefore the femoral canal is larger and it is for this reason that femoral hernia occurs more frequently in women.

The femoral canal. Lying beneath the inguinal ligament is a tube of fascia known as the femoral sheath and formed from the transver-salis fascia and the fascia covering the iliacus muscle. The sheath contains the femoral artery and vein and at its medial part there is a small gap 1·25 cm in length, just large enough to admit the tip of the little finger; this is the femoral canal. Beside the femoral sheath is the femoral nerve; all of these structures together with the deep inguinal lymph nodes are contained in an area known as the femoral triangle.

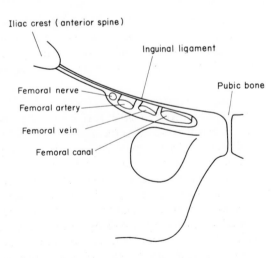

Fig. 75. *Contents of the femoral triangle.*

The femoral canal provides a pathway for the lymphatic vessels from the lower limb to the external iliac nodes, as well as allowing for expansion of the femoral vein. The neck of the femoral canal is narrow, hence a hernia occurring here may well be irreducible and often strangulates.

Features of femoral hernia. This type of hernia is very rare in children but may occur from about the age of twenty onwards. Symptoms are far less evident than those of inguinal hernia; many patients may only notice a small swelling which they tend to ignore for possibly years until one day strangulation occurs. The hernial sac is narrow as it passes through the femoral canal but once it is released it may curve in an upward direction and expand considerably into the loose tissues of the groin—this may cause the bulk of the hernia to lie above the level of the inguinal ligament. In order to arrive at a correct differential diagnosis the neck of the hernia must be examined; in the inguinal hernia this lies above the line of the inguinal ligament, whilst in the femoral hernia it lies below.

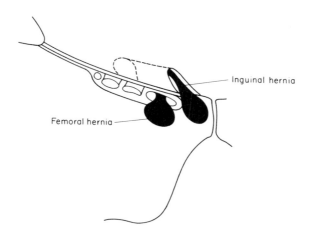

Fig. 76. *Sites of inguinal and femoral herniae.*

Treatment of femoral hernia. Surgery is the only effective treatment and should be undertaken so as to reduce the possibility of strangulation. A truss is of no value for this type of hernia. Herniorrhaphy is performed, for which there are several techniques, but the main features of this operation are to replace the contents of the hernial sac in the abdomen through an incision either above or below the inguinal ligament, and having ligated the now empty hernial sac this too can be drawn back through the femoral canal which is closed over it.

Strangulated femoral hernia

This occurs because the femoral canal is narrow and does not allow the hernia to be reduced. The length of gut involved in the hernia may also become gangrenous. When the hernial sac is incised at operation care must be taken with the removal of the bloodstained fluid it contains. The neck of the sac may require stretching in order to release the contents and this may be followed by resection and anastomosis of the loop of gut.

Umbilical hernia

Exomphalos

Exomphalos is the most severe form of umbilical hernia and occurs about one in six thousand births. It is due to the failure of all or part of the midgut to return to the abdominal cavity during early

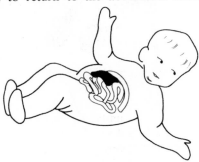

Fig. 77. *Exomphalos.*

development of the fetus (*see* Chapter 8). Covering the abdominal contents is a very thin walled hernial sac composed only of the amniotic membrane, Wharton's jelly and peritoneum; this is likely to rupture during birth. The contents of the hernia may be the small and large intestine and the liver. A minor type of exomphalos may be present in which a loop of small intestine or a Meckel's diverticulum is present in the base of the umbilical cord which is attached to it; for this reason the midwife always carefully inspects the base of the cord before applying a clamp.

Treatment. The birth of a baby with this severe abnormality necessitates very skilled and prompt surgery within a few hours of birth. Adjacent tissues are mobilized to form flaps as a covering for the organs in order to enclose them in the abdominal cavity. This condition carries a high mortality rate.

Umbilical hernia in children

This occurs with equal incidence in both sexes and consists of a herniation through a weak umbilical scar. It is rare for gut contained in the hernial sac to strangulate or perforate. The hernia is often only apparent when it increases in size when the child cries. There may be some enlargement during the early weeks of life but this is followed by gradual and spontaneous return to normal over several months or even years.

Treatment. On the whole no treatment is indicated unless the hernia persists until the child is nine or ten years old, when surgical repair may be undertaken. The use of adhesive strapping or similar abdominal binders have proved ineffective.

Para-umbilical hernia in adults

This condition is not a true umbilical hernia because it does not herniate through the umbilical scar but through the linea alba just above the umbilicus and therefore the hernia is in close proximity to it. The hernial sac is formed of the greater omentum and contains small intestine and occasionally part of the transverse colon. As the hernia enlarges it has a tendency to become pendulous. This type of hernia is more common in women aged between thirty-five and fifty years who are obese and have lax abdominal muscles following repeated pregnancies. The sheer weight of the hernia may cause a dragging pain and gastrointestinal symptoms are common with occasional attacks of intestinal colic.

Treatment. Surgical treatment is indicated as the hernia may strangulate. Prior to operation the patient should endeavour to lose weight. The intestine is returned to the abdomen, the hernial sac is removed and then the abdominal wall strengthened either by suturing or possibly with the use of strips of fascia (these may be taken from the thigh).

Incisional hernia
This type of hernia usually occurs in a laparotomy wound starting as a swelling along the line of the scar which increases in size until the contents can no longer be reduced. If the overlying scar tissue is very thin then peristaltic waves may be seen. Attacks of subacute intestinal obstruction are common and the hernia may strangulate. Predisposing factors to the formation of an incisional hernia are obesity, chronic cough and any infection in the vicinity of the wound, for example peritonitis.

Treatment. Surgical repair is necessary and by one of several techniques the contents of the hernial sac are replaced in the abdomen and the scar strengthened; this may be by the use of non-absorbable sutures, Dacron net or other suitable materials.

Nursing care in hernia. It has been seen that surgery is required for treatment of most types of hernia, and as obesity and chronic cough are two of the chief predisposing factors it is important that they are dealt with prior to operation. The patient who is awaiting admission to hospital for herniorrhaphy may benefit from dietary advice and possibly treatment of any respiratory infection. Smoking should be discouraged for at least two weeks prior to operation. The pre-operative care as described in Chapter 1 should be carried out and in addition the patient will require the abdomen and pubic area to be shaved, and abdominal and breathing exercises to be taught by the physiotherapist. No other specific preparation is necessary unless it is intended to repair the hernia with strips of fascia in which case one leg should be prepared by shaving from the thigh to below the knee.

Following herniotomy the amount of pain experienced is minimal and the patient will probably be mobile again very quickly. When a herniorrhaphy or hernioplasty has been carried out it is likely to prove more painful and there is lack of movement of the abdominal wall to aid respiratory movements and coughing; it is important therefore to encourage deep breathing exercises. It is usual to start exercises of the abdominal muscles on about the third or fourth post-operative day. The patient is got up out of bed for a short period on the day following operation, but this may be delayed for several days if the operation was to repair a large incisional hernia. Retention of urine is a common complication following operation for hernia and may be relieved by carbachol 250–500 microgrammes by subcutaneous injection or 1–4 mg orally. It is important to observe the urine as a stitch inadvertently passed through the bladder wall may cause haematuria which will require treatment by catheterization and continuous drainage of the bladder. When the patient is fit and able to be discharged from hospital about twelve days after operation he should be encouraged to have a period of convalescence before resuming work; this should be for as long as six weeks if he is returning to manual work that involves lifting, but may be only about two weeks if he has a sedentary occupation. Provided the pre- and post-operative period has been free from complications the patient may be discharged home as early as forty-eight hours after operation, in which case the nurse must make sure that the community health team has been advised.

Nursing care in strangulated hernia. This condition requires an emergency operation to relieve the pressure on the gut hopefully before it becomes gangrenous. Relief of the severe pain will need to be undertaken and the stomach contents aspirated through a Ryle's tube which is left in place. The patient is likely to be dehydrated and this must be corrected by the giving of intravenous fluids, and a sample of blood will be taken for electrolyte estimation and any deficiencies corrected. During operation it may be necessary to resect an area of gut and carry out an anastomosis, but whether this has been done or not there is considerable risk of peritonitis developing; for this reason a broad spectrum antibiotic will be given. Aspiration of gastric contents will be continued until peristalsis and bowel sounds return. The remainder of the postoperative care follows that for repair of an uncomplicated hernia, and the patient should be advised a period of convalescence.

CHAPTER 12

Intestinal Obstruction

Intestinal obstruction may occur at any age in life and is precipitated by a variety of factors; it is generally considered as being one of three types namely, acute, subacute or chronic.

Acute intestinal obstruction
Causes

(1) Occlusion of the bowel preventing onward movement of the gut contents. This may be due to actual blockage of the lumen by such objects as gall stones or foreign bodies, disease processes affecting the wall of the gut as is found in regional ileitis and neoplasms, and finally pressure from outside the gut caused by adhesions, inflammation, fibrous bands and neoplasms.

(2) Strangulation of the bowel may occur when there is interference with the blood supply to a part. This is found to be the cause in such conditions as intussusception, volvulus, hernia or bands of adhesions.

(3) Paralysis of a length of intestine as found in the condition of paralytic ileus, here there is no gross lesion responsible but interference with the nerve supply to the gut reduces its ability to carry out normal peristaltic movements.

Clinical features
Intestinal obstruction gives rise to certain features although not all of them need be present in order to confirm the diagnosis, i.e.

(1) Intestinal colic. The pain is felt mainly around the umbilicus

and may be severe. It tends to occur in attacks with painfree intervals between.

(2) Vomiting. At first this is of partly digested food followed later by bile stained fluid, and finally a black/brown fluid with an unpleasant odour due to the altered blood it contains—the so-called 'faecal vomit'. The time of onset of vomiting gives some indication as to the level at which the obstruction occurs: if this is high in the gastrointestinal tract then vomiting will be an early feature, whereas for a low obstruction vomiting will not occur until later.

(3) Constipation. This is termed 'absolute' because once the lower bowel has emptied there is no passage of either faeces or flatus.

(4) Abdominal distension. This feature occurs mainly when obstruction is low in the tract; visible peristalsis may also be seen.

Diagnosis
A diagnosis of intestinal obstruction may be reached at the conclusion of a full clinical examination. The doctor may request the taking of a plain X-ray of the abdomen for which the patient is sat upright. The X-ray film will show loops of gut distended with gas, and also the presence of fluid levels; the latter may appear within three or four hours of the obstruction occurring.

Principles of treatment
To relieve the situation three main types of treatment are required:

(1) Aspiration of gastrointestinal contents may be carried out satisfactorily through a Ryle's tube passed into the stomach, aspiration taking place at regular intervals for several hours before surgery is undertaken. If the gut has become strangulated then surgery is urgent but prior to this a Miller–Abbott type tube is passed into the intestine so that fluid proximal to the obstruction may be aspirated. This tube is 1·75 m in length and has a double lumen, one is used for aspiration of fluid and the other is connected to a balloon at the end which is inflated with air or water which encourages the passage of the tube on through the pylorus into the small intestine. At the other end the two outlets of the double lumen

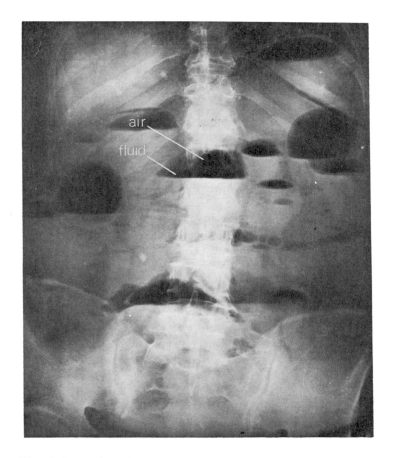

Fig. 78. *X-ray of gut showing gas and fluid levels in intestinal obstruction.*

tube are labelled 'suction' and 'filling'. If the tube fails to travel far along the gut it may be removed later by pulling it out through the nostril, on the other hand if it has been carried some way by peristalsis the outlets are cut off and the tube allowed to continue its journey through the entire gut (*see* Fig. 5, p. 17).

(2) Fluid replacement. Large quantities of digestive fluids continue to be secreted into the lumen of the gut and fail to be reabsorbed in their usual manner because of the obstruction. This fluid amounts to about eight litres per day, of which four litres are produced above the level of the pylorus and about four litres below. Accumulation of the fluid leads to vomiting, and whether this occurs or the fluid is aspirated the body loses valuable sodium, potassium and chloride ions. The loss of potassium may increase the possibility of paralytic ileus occurring. All output must be measured (vomit, aspirate and urine) and then this loss made good by the administration of fluid by the intravenous route. Isotonic saline (normal saline 0·9%) may be given at first, followed by dextrose/saline (dextrose 4·3% and saline 0·18%) as maintenance therapy. The amount given must be sufficient to replace the initial loss and then to maintain normal hydration by infusing an additional three litres of fluid per twenty-four hours. The daily requirements of an adult will be about 6 g sodium chloride (104 mmol) and 4 g potassium (60 mmol). It is important that a sample of blood is taken to estimate the electrolyte levels, haemoglobin, plasma proteins and haematocrit before the commencement of the infusion. The infusion may need to be continued for several days and therefore additional vitamins especially B and C should be given, which can be in the form of Parenterovite 2 ampoules to each litre of fluid infused.

(3) Surgical relief of the obstruction. One of a number of operations may be carried out the aim being to relieve the obstruction and maintain the viability of the gut if at all possible. Decompression of the gut may be necessary before resection and end-to-end anastomosis is performed. The exception to this form of treatment is paralytic ileus which may complicate surgery of the gut and be relieved by gastric aspiration and fluid replacement.

Acute intestinal obstruction in babies

Obstruction may be present at birth in which case one of a number of congenital anomalies may be responsible.

Atresia and stenosis

This condition may occur in the duodenum, jejunum or ileum with a frequency of one in five thousand live births. Atresia may be such that the lumen of the intestine is obstructed by a septum (Type I) or a segment of gut appears as a fibrous cord (Type II) or the two blind ends of gut are quite separate (Type III). In the proximal part of the gut peristalsis continues, the wall becomes hypertrophied and the

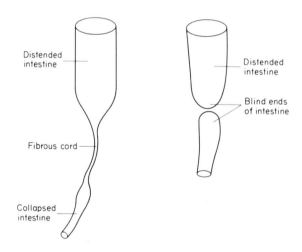

Fig. 79. *Intestinal atresia in newborn.*

intestine grossly dilated. Eventually, the circulation is impaired and this progresses to necrosis of the gut and perforation. The intestine beyond the obstruction may contain meconium and very viscid mucus. Diagnosis is assisted by taking an abdominal X-ray, and treatment consists of gastric aspiration and correction of electrolyte imbalance by the administration of intravenous fluids. Surgery is required urgently so that the affected segment of intestine can be resected and an anastomosis carried out.

Malrotation

Failure of the embryonic gut to complete its rotation (*see* Chapter 4) may cause the upper small intestine to occupy the right side of the abdomen whilst the caecum and colon are on the left side. This arrangement may predispose to the formation of adhesive bands which can cause obstruction. If a mesenteric pedicle twists it forms a volvulus of the intestine causing strangulation of the gut and will give rise to similar features as for malrotation with the addition of blood being passed per rectum. Diagnosis may be assisted by X-ray of the abdomen; air introduced into the stomach can act as a contrast medium. Surgical treatment is required to correct this condition.

Meconium ileus

This is present at birth and is associated with fibrocystic disease of the pancreas (*see* Chapter 7). The pancreatic juice is deficient in an enzyme which causes the contents of the small intestine to be thick, grey and like putty in appearance. This condition predisposes to intestinal obstruction occurring within a few days of birth. If unrelieved volvulus may occur or the gut may perforate causing meconium peritonitis. Surgical treatment is necessary to remove the sticky contents of the gut, and maybe perform a resection and anastomosis of the intestine. Treatment of the underlying fibrocystic disease is necessary to prevent recurrence.

Imperforate anus

This condition has been described in Chapter 9.

Hirschsprung's disease

This condition has been described in Chapter 9.

Features of obstruction in the newborn. Vomiting is often the first sign that presents in this situation and occurs within twenty-four hours of birth. It will be noted that the baby fails to pass meconium and as time progresses the abdomen is seen to become more distended.

Diagnosis and treatment. The same principles of diagnosis apply to babies as adults, namely a plain abdominal X-ray with the patient in the erect position so that gas and fluid levels can be seen. The nurse may be required to hold the baby and will require a lead apron or shield for her own protection. Following diagnosis, the stomach must be emptied, an intravenous infusion commenced so that electrolytes can be replaced and hydration maintained prior to surgical correction of the anomaly. Congenital anomalies in the gut may be only one of a number of such conditions present and therefore a detailed examination must be made and the most appropriate form of treatment embarked upon.

Intussusception

This condition is likely to occur in male babies between the age of six and eighteen months, and may result from a change in diet at weaning or follow a virus infection where the lymphoid tissue in the gut has become enlarged. The terminal ileum becomes invaginated into the colon causing intestinal obstruction and leading to gangrene of the invaginated part. Intussusception causes acute and sudden episodes of abdominal pain which makes the baby draw up his legs and scream. Attacks of pain recur at about half-hourly intervals at first, but later the painfree intervals become shorter. Vomiting occurs and the baby passes stools of bright red blood and mucus—the so-called 'red currant jelly' stools.

Diagnosis. On abdominal examination a sausage-shaped tumour may be palpable, and the condition is confirmed by performing a barium enema and noting the obstruction on the X-ray film.

Treatment. The baby will quickly become dehydrated and so replacement of fluid by the intravenous route is necessary, and electrolyte imbalance corrected. A tube should be passed and the stomach aspirated. If a diagnosis has been made promptly it may be possible to reduce the intussusception by hydrostatic pressure. The baby is anaesthetized, and a Foley catheter introduced into the rectum and the bag inflated. Barium sulphate is run from a height of one metre above the operating table and the progress observed by fluoroscopy. This is carried out for forty-five minutes and should continue only if progress is being made. Where diagnosis is not made until later it will be necessary to perform an exploratory laparotomy and reduce the intussusception. The bowel may be sutured to the peritoneum to prevent a recurrence. If the viability of the gut is in doubt it should be resected and anastomosed. In intussusception there is a recurrence rate of between 1 and 3%.

Acute intestinal obstruction in adults

Acute intestinal obstruction may occur at any age in adults and results from a number of causes. These include:

Strangulated hernia
This is more likely to be an indirect inguinal hernia in men or a femoral hernia in women. Strangulated herniae account for about 50% of all cases of intestinal obstruction. Diagnosis can be made on physical examination. Treatment is surgical and should be carried out with the minimum of delay.

Adhesions
Adhesions and bands may result after abdominal surgery and peritonitis. Surgical treatment may only partially relieve the situation and recurrence is likely.

Volvulus
This condition occurs at both extremes of life, the newborn and the elderly. In the latter, the pelvic colon twists (*see* Fig. 8) and in so

doing interferes with the blood passing through the mesentery to supply it. Volvulus in adults occurs more often in those taking a vegetarian diet where there is more bulk in the food residues. When the condition occurs it causes sudden and severe abdominal pain,

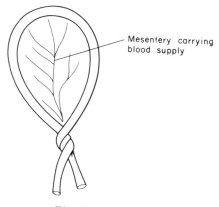

Mesentery carrying blood supply

Fig. 80. *Volvulus*.

accompanied by vomiting, constipation and increasing abdominal distension. No flatus is passed. Diagnosis is made by palpating a tense swelling in the pelvis, and observing a large gas shadow on the left side of the abdomen following the taking of a plain X-ray. The volvulus may be relieved by guiding a flatus tube through the twisted gut under direct sigmoidoscopy followed by resection of the affected area of the gut later if necessary. If this treatment is unsuccessful then laparotomy will be necessary so that the volvulus can be reduced and deflated prior to resection and anastomosis.

Mesenteric embolus and thrombosis

Emboli may occur in the mesenteric arteries as a complication of myocardial infarction and bacterial endocarditis although these are relatively infrequent. The superior mesenteric artery may also be affected by atheroma. Portal pyaemia and cirrhosis of the liver may also predispose to thrombus formation in the mesenteric veins.

Whether the occlusion to the blood supply of the intestine be either in the arteries or the veins it causes infarction of the gut wall tissue and obstruction results. The patient collapses with the sudden severe abdominal colic, passes blood per rectum, and suffers from shock. Surgical treatment is required which may take the form of

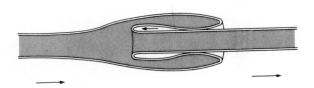

Fig. 81. *Intussusception.*

resection and anastomosis of the intestine, possibly preceded and followed by the administration of heparin, or either embolectomy, endarterectomy or a by-pass graft. The patient is in urgent need of fluid replacement to correct the shock.

Paralytic ileus
This condition may occur as a post-operative complication following abdominal surgery and peritonitis or result from severe electrolyte disturbance, intestinal disorders such as ulcerative colitis and typhoid fever, or the action of hypotensive agents such as the anticholinergic and ganglion-blocking drugs. Paralytic ileus results when there is absence of motor activity in the gut and therefore no peristalsis. The intestine dilates and the patient exhibits all the features of acute intestinal obstruction. No bowel sounds are heard on auscultation. Treatment of the cause of paralytic ileus together with gastric aspiration and correction of electrolyte imbalance by the administration of intravenous fluids should be carried out. If the cause is due to an excess of hypotensive drugs then prostigmine 1 mg intramuscularly may be given as an antidote with effect.

Subacute or chronic intestinal obstruction

Chronic disorders of the bowel may result in a subacute or chronic form of intestinal obstruction, and the latter type frequently become acute. Such bowel disorders may be regional ileitis, ulcerative colitis or carcinoma of the colon. The patient experiences alternating episodes of diarrhoea and constipation accompanied by abdominal distension and colicky pain. On plain X-ray of the abdomen dilated loops of gut with fluid levels will be seen. Treatment is directed to that of the underlying cause and may necessitate surgery.

Peritonitis

This is an inflammatory reaction occurring on the serous membranes which form the peritoneum and line the peritoneal cavity.

The peritoneal cavity extends from under the diaphragm to the pelvis, and from the anterior to the posterior abdominal walls. This cavity is lined by a serous membrane which is derived from the endothelial lining of the main body cavity in the embryo and eventually divides to form two distinct membranes—the pleura and the peritoneum. The peritoneum becomes invaginated by the ingrowing of the abdominal organs and thus forms two layers, a parietal and visceral layer. In the male the peritoneal cavity is closed, but in the female it is in communication with the exterior by means of the open ends of the uterine tubes. The position of the peritoneum can best be considered by tracing its points of attachment in the body cavity. Starting at the umbilicus, the parietal layer can be traced upwards to the undersurface of the diaphragm as far as the upper and lower coronary ligaments of the liver where it is reflected back over the liver (leaving an area uncovered which is the bare area of the liver), encloses the liver and descends from the porta hepatis as a double sheet (lesser omentum) to the lesser curvature of the stomach. The peritoneum divides to enclose the stomach,

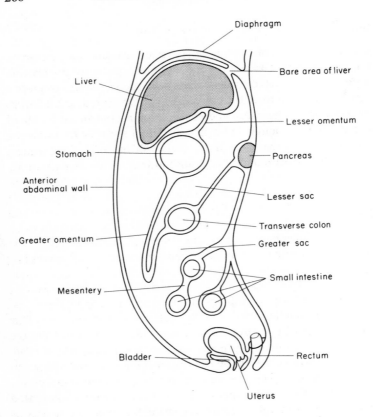

Fig. 82. *The peritoneal cavity.*

rejoins at the greater curvature and then loops down into the
abdomen, turns on itself (greater omentum) and passes back to
become attached along the length of the transverse colon, rejoins
and passes to the posterior abdominal wall. The peritoneum then
divides to cover the anterior aspect of the pancreas; the upper part
passing up the posterior abdominal wall to the bare area of the liver
is reflected back over the liver as far as the porta hepatis. The other
part of the peritoneum passes down the posterior abdominal wall,

enclosing loops of intestine as it passes to cover the pelvic viscera and subsequently continues up the anterior abdominal wall to the umbilicus as the parietal layer. The part of the peritoneum which encloses the loops of small intestine whilst remaining attached to the posterior abdominal wall is called the mesentery which forms a supporting tissue to the blood vessels and lymphatics which supply the gut. The arrangement of the peritoneum causes the formation of two cavities although these are in communication through the foramen of Winslow, the lesser sac is situated behind the lesser omentum and between the stomach and liver, whilst the remainder forms the main peritoneal cavity or greater sac. It will be noted that such organs as the kidneys, duodenum, pancreas and major blood vessels are only covered on their anterior aspect by peritoneum and therefore remain outside the peritoneal cavity and are said to be retroperitoneal. The folds of the peritoneum together with the attachments for the liver cause the formation of potential spaces just under the diaphragm. There are five main subphrenic spaces which become clinically important when filled with pus giving rise to a subphrenic abscess.

Causes of peritonitis: may be divided into two external causes which may result from infection introduced along the track of a penetrating wound; internal causes which originate from perforation of a peptic ulcer, appendix or other organ, by direct spread from infection in the female genital tract, or by blood borne spread from infections elsewhere in the body. The latter cause may result from lobar pneumonia which gives rise to a pneumococcal peritonitis, or other respiratory tract infection leading to streptococcal peritonitis. Most cases of peritonitis are as a result of heavy contamination of the peritoneal cavity following rupture of an organ. Infection may become localized, forming an abscess which can be drained, otherwise infection is diffuse and gives rise to general peritonitis. When the peritoneum is inflamed it becomes congested and produces a large amount of exudate which covers over the parietal peritoneum. This fluid becomes purulent, causes the intestine to become paralysed (paralytic ileus) and if untreated may lead to death of the patient. The fact that the positions of the mesentery and colon divide the peritoneal cavity into four main spaces helps to confine the inflammatory exudate in one area when acute infection occurs.

Clinical features. The onset of peritonitis may be gradual, or sudden if it occurs as a result of perforation of a peptic ulcer. Abdominal pain is experienced when the parietal peritoneum is affected as this layer shares the same nerve supply as the area of abdominal wall under which it lies. Characteristically, the patient lies still in bed with the knees drawn up towards the chest, and appears pale with an anxious facial expression and sunken eyes. Vomiting and constipation are present. When paralytic ileus develops the abdomen is distended, rigid and tender. The infection may become localized and then a mass which is tender on abdominal palpation will be found. Observations of the temperature and pulse will show both to be raised, but the blood pressure is likely to be lowered due to the loss of plasma into the peritoneal exudate.

Treatment and nursing care. Usually surgery is indicated in the form of a laparotomy in order to drain the peritoneum, but this is only one aspect of the treatment ordered. The patient may be nursed with the head of the bed raised to allow drainage of purulent material towards the pelvis. Nothing is given by mouth and hydration is maintained by an intravenous infusion to which electrolytes are added if required as a result of blood taken for testing. A blood or plasma transfusion may be necessary. A broad spectrum antibiotic will be prescribed. It is important to empty the stomach of its contents and a nasogastric tube will be passed for this purpose and aspirated at intervals. This patient is ill and in considerable pain and therefore will require skilled nursing which must include a change of position in order to relieve pressure, care of the skin and a renewal of bed linen and nightclothes. Frequent oral hygiene is necessary. Observations of temperature, pulse and respiration rates will be taken and recorded four hourly, together with a fluid intake and urine output balance chart. If the peritoneal cavity has been drained then renewal of the dressing will be required, or attention to the vacuum drainage container if this type is in use. The physiotherapist will encourage exercise of the limbs and also deep breathing to prevent further complications. When the patient shows improvement and bowel sounds are heard then small quantities of fluid by mouth will be allowed and the interval increased between gastric aspiration. When a satisfactory fluid intake is achieved the infusion will be discontinued and small light meals introduced. By this stage the patient should be more mobile and given every encouragement in this respect. The amount of peritoneal drainage will be less and the drainage tube can be shortened and finally removed, the area being covered by a dry dressing which is renewed when necessary. If the infection becomes localized and an abscess forms this can be incised and drained, the foregoing treatment and nursing care applies equally to this situation.

Associated conditions of the peritoneum

Subphrenic abscess

In this condition pus is present under the diaphragm and may result from infection in the gall bladder or pancreas or perforation of the stomach or duodenum. The onset may be insidious, the patient experiencing abdominal and chest pain, often with hiccough. A pleural effusion and pyrexia may be present. Diagnosis is confirmed by taking an X-ray, and the treatment involves the administration of antibiotics together with incision and drainage of the abscess.

Tuberculous mesenteric lymphadenitis and peritonitis

Tuberculous infection in the mesenteric lymph nodes is usually of the bovine type which is acquired by drinking infected milk. There may be pyrexia, loss of weight and abdominal pain. On X-ray the glands appear to be calcified. Tuberculous peritonitis is of two types, one which gives rise to gross ascites when the bacilli can be isolated from the ascitic fluid, and the other when the peritoneal surfaces become adherent with the fibrinous exudate resulting in intestinal obstruction. Antituberculous drugs are used to treat all these conditions.

Tumours

Primary tumours of the peritoneum are rare but secondary ones are common and usually result from a primary carcinoma elsewhere which gives rise to the formation of nodules or extensive adhesions by spread across the peritoneal membrane. Ascites is common. Chemotherapy in the form of cytotoxic drugs may be prescribed. Paracentesis abdominis may be carried out but this usually only gives short-term relief.

Haemoperitoneum

Blood in the peritoneal cavity may result from trauma or occur spontaneously as a result of a ruptured ovarian cyst, uterine tube or spleen or be due to acute pancreatitis. The blood loss may be gradual or sudden: if the latter then it is likely to be severe giving rise to acute abdominal pain, rigidity and collapse of the patient. This constitutes an acute abdominal emergency, the patient requiring urgent resuscitative measures and an exploratory laparotomy.

Torsion of the omentum

This is more likely to occur in obese and middle-aged ladies, as a result of adhesions to the parietal peritoneum. The mesenteric veins are occluded and strangulation of the gut occurs. The patient experiences sudden, severe abdominal pain with marked tenderness and rigidity above the affected area of gut. This is accompanied by nausea and vomiting. Surgical treatment is necessary which takes the form of an exploratory laparotomy with resection and anastomosis of the twisted segment of gut.

CHAPTER 13

Paediatric Nursing

Throughout this book paediatric conditions of the gastrointestinal tract have been described in the appropriate chapters; in this section some of the general features of these conditions together with the tests and investigations which may assist in their diagnosis will be considered along with the general nursing care of the baby and young child. The adult patient and older child are able to give a history of their illness and report any change in the character of the pain experienced, whereas for the baby and toddler the nurse must observe and as far as possible interpret any change she may notice in the way the baby lies, cries or takes his feeds, besides other more routine observations. The nurse is helped in this task by the baby's mother who can give a history of the condition before admission to hospital became necessary, and providing she is allowed and encouraged to share in the care of her baby in the ward will report any unfamiliar signs she may notice.

SIGNS AND SYMBOLS

Abdominal pain
Recurring attacks of abdominal pain are common in young children and although there may be some organic cause very often this is not so and the problem is an emotional one. Sensible parents will be aware of this and deal satisfactorily with the situation, but where the

273

parents have little insight then the doctor has to try and help both age groups. It is important that investigations are carried out to eliminate an organic cause, and then psychotherapy may be needed. This condition usually occurs in children between the ages of four and thirteen years, pain being complained of after breakfast and regarded by some as being an indication of not wanting to go to school. Headache may also be present. Often there are behavioural disturbances and the problem may be due to difficult family relationships between the patient and his parents or his brothers and sisters. Conflict between the parents may also produce this type of reaction in the children. In some cases both an organic and emotional factor may be causing the pain, improvement may be seen when the cause has been treated, and again the child psychologist may assist in this recovery.

For the very young child who cannot communicate verbally the nurse must observe the way the baby draws up his legs and cries when attacks of abdominal pain occur, or whether he dislikes being moved or handled.

Vomiting

Vomiting in young children may be due to a variety of causes, these include:

Dietetic causes
Underfeeding in the newborn is probably the most common cause, and in this case the vomit is of milk and milk curds. The hungry baby will cry continually, during which time he swallows quantities of air, and when the feed is offered it is gulped down hungrily and then vomited whilst bringing up wind. This situation, together with observation of the small frequent stools and the failure to gain weight should alert the nurse to increasing the baby's diet. An allergy to milk or a congenital intolerance to lactose are occasionally found in young babies and will encourage vomiting of feeds.

Infections
Infection in the gastrointestinal tract will generally cause vomiting

of food with mucus and sometimes blood, and this is often accompanied by colicky type abdominal pain. In young children infections in other systems often cause vomiting, and this feature may be the first clue to the fact that the child is unwell. Tonsillitis, otitis media and infections in the central nervous system, urinary or respiratory tracts cause the baby to vomit food and gastric juices which may lead to dehydration. For the child with pertussis (whooping cough) the vomiting of mucus and some food often occurs after an attack of coughing. Some antibiotics which may be used in the treatment of infections may also induce vomiting and may need to be given by injection at first.

Anatomical disorders of the gastrointestinal tract

Obstruction to the passage of food through the tract will cause vomiting (see Chapter 12) which may be forceful and described as projectile, the vomit landing a metre or so away from the baby. Non-obstructive causes such as a hiatus hernia will cause the baby to vomit a recently taken food, together with mucus and sometimes a little blood. Treatment of the underlying cause is required for all these conditions.

Metabolic causes

Of the metabolic causes probably phenylketonuria and galacto-saemia are the most likely. Investigation will be necessary and then treatment with the appropriate diet should bring about an improvement in the condition.

Cerebral conditions

Cerebral injury which may result from birth trauma, or the existence of raised intracranial pressure due to a space-occupying lesion or hydrocephalus may cause the baby to vomit the stomach contents in a projectile manner without warning.

Endocrine disorders

Endocrine disorders may not be apparent until the child is older, but if adrenal hyperplasia is present at birth this may cause vomiting.

Severe systemic conditions

Conditions such as uraemia and malignant neoplasms may cause the child to vomit very fluid gastric contents. This usually occurs in the terminal stages of the illness.

Types of stools

Normal stools

The nurse must be able to recognize a normal stool from a baby in order that she can detect and report an abnormal one if it occurs; the nurse should make a habit of observing all bowel actions before she discards them. During the first one to three days of life the baby passes a tarry, greenish–black semisolid stool called meconium on about three occasions each day. The stool then changes to being soft and a greenish–brown colour for about the third and fourth days, and is known as the changing stool. From about the fifth day the stools change again, the breast fed baby passes a soft mustard yellow stool maybe on five or six occasions each day, whilst the baby which is fed on cows' milk passes a semiformed and bulky pale yellow–grey stool perhaps four or five times a day. Great variation in the size and number of stools passed occurs in normal healthy breast and artificially fed infants, and the mother must be reassured in this respect. Some breast fed infants pass one large bright yellow stool on alternate days or even at longer intervals and thrive normally. On the whole the baby fed on cows' milk passes less stools than the breast fed baby and also has a tendency to constipation; this rarely if ever happens to a baby fed on breast milk. When mixed feeding is introduced the stools change to being formed and brown and usually one or two each day.

Abnormal stools

For the baby that is underfed the stools become small, frequent and dark green in colour, they are acid in reaction and have a sour odour. Mucus and bile may be present. If overfeeding is present then bright green, offensive and frothy stools may be passed very frequently. These stools are very acid and contain quantities of unwanted fat and carbohydrate. Infection in the gastrointestinal tract gives rise to the frequent passing of bright green, offensive fluid stools, which may contain partially digested food and mucus. Blood may be present in the form of melaena as a result of swallowing blood or bleeding from along the gastrointestinal tract. The stools are usually soft and tarry black in appearance. Fresh blood may be present when bleeding occurs from an anal fissure or rectal polyp and the stool may be normal, soft or hard according to the cause.

Constipation

Infrequent stools are not harmful to the child provided they remain soft and are passed without discomfort. Parents and nurses must appreciate that great variation occurs with regard to the number of times defaecation occurs either each day or week, and what appears as a normal pattern for one healthy child in a family may differ considerably from that of its healthy brother or sister. Many children are subjected to considerable psychological and physical trauma because parents insist on a daily bowel action and may give aperients unnecessarily in order to achieve this; on the other hand training the child to empty the bowel when the occasion arises contributes to good habit formation and may help reduce the likelihood of disorders occurring in later years. Where true constipation exists, the child passes hard, dry faeces accompanied by considerable pain. This may be due in the newborn to underfeeding and can often be easily remedied by the addition of a little extra sugar and water to the feeds. Constipation is a feature of congenital anomalies in the gut such as intestinal atresia or Hirschsprung's disease. Local conditions such as an anal fissure may prevent the child from defaecating when necessary and so aggravate the situation. Severe systemic conditions such as nephritis, tuberculosis and meningitis may all be accompanied by constipation. Psychological factors mainly as a result of faulty habit training are an additional cause. Treatment of constipation is aimed at the underlying cause, but occasionally an aperient is needed until a normal pattern of bowel actions is re-established. Suitable aperients for young children include compound syrup of figs 2·5–10 ml orally, magnesium hydroxide mixture (Milk or Cream of Magnesia) 5–10 ml orally, or Senokot half a tablet or half a teaspoon of granules orally.

AIDS TO DIAGNOSIS

Oesophagoscopy
This investigation may be carried out to detect oesophagitis in conditions of dysphagia or where there is gastro-oesophageal reflux. A general anaesthetic is given and an endotracheal tube passed. A fibrescope or Negus oesophagoscope is used.

Biopsy of the small intestine
This investigation will be necessary in malabsorption disorders. For children under one year of age a paediatric version of the Crosby capsule can be used, for all other children the adult type is suitable (*see* Chapter 8). The procedure is usually carried out in the morning and apart from not giving the child breakfast no other preparation is necessary. If the child is likely to be cooperative and not pull on the polythene tube then they may be up and about in the ward, but if the child is nervous then they are best given a sedative and kept in bed. Once the capsule has been swallowed its progress through the gut can be followed by fluoroscopy; it should reach the small intestine in about two hours. The biopsy is then taken and the capsule removed. Very occasionally haemorrhage complicates this procedure.

Fat absorption tests
All dietary fat is almost entirely absorbed by the gut, that present in the faeces is as a result of bacterial synthesis together with desquamated intestinal cells. Normally in healthy children the daily fat content of the faeces does not exceed 3 g, therefore for the majority of cases it is sufficient to collect the total faeces passed for three consecutive days whilst the child takes a normal diet. Where more precise investigation is required then the child is fed a known

quantity of fat over a period of five days during which time all stools are saved for fat estimation.

D-*xylose absorption test*

This test is used to help diagnose defects in the intestinal mucosa which are not attributed to the malabsorption syndrome. D-xylose is a sugar not normally present in the diet or in blood, and is actively absorbed in the upper part of the jejunum. An oral dose of 5 g is given, and in the normal child 65% of this is rapidly absorbed, and of that amount 40% is excreted in the urine. In normal circumstances more than 25% of that excreted in the urine occurs within five hours of administration of the sugar. If the urine is collected over a period of twenty-four hours, then the whole amount absorbed should be recovered from the urine. This investigation is of no value where there is renal disease.

Sigmoidoscopy

This investigation should be carried out as a matter of routine where any dysfunction of the colon is suspected. No preparation is necessary, the child should not be given an enema as this may make for a state of non-cooperation and also damage the mucosa further. Just occasionally it may be necessary to give a small rectal washout using saline. If the child will cooperate with the doctor then a general anaesthetic need not be given, but if the child is anxious and easily frightened then it is preferable to give an anaesthetic. For a baby up to a few months old a small paediatric sigmoidoscope is used, but after that age the adult instrument can be safely used. A biopsy of the mucosa is taken through the sigmoidoscope. The whole procedure should last only a few minutes.

PAEDIATRIC NURSING PROCEDURES

Gastric lavage

This procedure may be necessary prior to operation or simply to remove excess mucus or milk curds from the baby's stomach in the early neonatal period.

Requirements:

Trolley or tray containing: glass or plastic saline funnel (120 ml); short length of tubing and tapered connection; straight catheter size 14 FG (7 EG); jug with measured amount of lotion (sterile water or normal saline) at 38°C; tray containing 10 ml syringe; litmus paper; gallipot; lubricant (water or glycerine); large bowl; protective plastic sheet.

Method

Two nurses are required for this procedure. The baby is wrapped up securely to restrain the arms and legs and is sat upright on one nurse's lap. The nurse holds the baby close to her and supports his head with one hand and holds the baby securely with the other. The plastic is draped over the baby and tucked under his chin. The other nurse washes her hands and assembles the apparatus. The catheter is measured against the baby from the bridge of the nose to the xiphisternum—this is the distance which roughly corresponds to that from the lips into the stomach. The catheter is lubricated and passed into the baby's mouth on top of the tongue, as the baby sucks it can be very gently guided down the oesophagus. When the required length has been swallowed, the tube must be checked that it has entered the stomach, the end of the catheter can be placed under water and any bubbling noted. An eruction of bubbles may occur as air escapes from the stomach, but rhythmical bubbling corresponding to the respiratory rate indicates that the tube is in the trachea and must be withdrawn. Gastric contents may be aspirated and tested with the litmus paper, but it is not always possible to obtain gastric juice for this purpose. Checking of the tube in the stomach should be carried out by a trained nurse. The lotion is then run into the funnel and allowed to flow to the end of the connection before being connected to the catheter. By raising or lowering the funnel the rate of flow of the fluid is controlled. When the fluid level is near the bottom of the funnel, the apparatus is lowered to allow the fluid and gastric contents to siphon back and then the funnel is inverted over the bowl. The procedure is repeated several times until the aspirate is clear then the catheter is pinched and withdrawn quickly. By allowing the fluid to siphon back into the funnel a check can be made on the amount of fluid returned, and at the end of the procedure this should be measured and recorded. Both nurses will observe the baby for any cyanosis or other adverse effect during the procedure.

Tube feeding

The same equipment as for gastric lavage is required, although some may prefer to pass a tube with a smaller lumen when giving a feed. In addition the feed should be in a bottle in a container of warm water to keep it at the required temperature. Any medicines to be given should be poured and checked immediately before commencing the feed. The procedure as for gastric lavage is followed as far as checking the tube in position in the stomach, then the feed is poured into the funnel allowed to pass to the end of the connection before attaching it to the catheter. When the level of the feed nears the base of the funnel then more is added. Medicines should be given in the middle of the feed sandwiched between the milk feed; they should not be left to the end or mixed with the entire feed as there is always a possibility that the whole quantity of fluid is not given. When the last of the feed has reached the base of the funnel then 15 ml of sterile water can be run in to clear the remaining feed from the catheter and ensure that if fluid spills into the trachea during the withdrawal of the tube it is non-irritant. When the last of the fluid passes the connection then the catheter is pinched and withdrawn. The baby should be sat up and allowed to bring up wind in the usual way before having the napkin changed and made comfortable in the cot. The amount of feed given, drugs and observations of bowel action and urine passed should be recorded on the treatment chart.

Stoma care

Occasionally it is necessary for a baby or young child to have either a temporary or permanent colostomy or a stoma for an ileal conduit. Similar appliances as used by adults are available for children (in a suitable size) and the management of the stoma is identical to that for adults (see Chapter 1). Young children with a

K

colostomy generally take this in their stride and can be taught to care for it themselves under supervision. The nurse must remember that the mother may not be so adaptable and she will need just as much support and encouragement as any adult faced with a similar situation.

General care. For the majority of babies and toddlers admitted to hospital for investigation or treatment of a gastrointestinal condition the nurse should endeavour to find out from the mother the daily routine and as far as possible continue in a similar way. Where a baby lacks routine this may have contributed to its illness, and here the nurse functions as a health educator towards the mother. Wherever possible the mother should be encouraged to spend as much of the day as is practicable in hospital sharing in the nursing of the baby, so that he receives his care and comfort from the one who normally does this for him. Where a mother is unable to be with her baby, perhaps by reason of living a long way from hospital or other children and members of the family to care for, she should not be made to feel as though she has neglected the baby and she should be given every help to enable her to visit as frequently as possible. An older child will also appreciate visits from other members of his family and friends. The daily routine of feeding, bathing, dressing and resting should be encouraged and where possible children should be allowed up and about in the ward and playroom wearing normal day clothes. For the older child who can manage alone in the toilet the nurse must check on personal hygiene and handwashing, as gastrointestinal infections can spread quickly round the occupants of a children's ward. Care of the teeth is important and the nurse should encourage the child to carry this out under supervision. If the child is not well enough to be out of bed he may be dressed and lie on top of the bed where he can have easy access to his toys. All children with gastrointestinal infections and small babies should be isolated in cubicles where possible, either for their own or other patient's safety. If the child has persistent vomiting then frequent mouthwashes will be appreciated. If diarrhoea is present this may cause excoriation of the buttocks and frequent washing with soap and water, drying thoroughly and the application of a barrier cream will be necessary. Great care must be exercised when removing soiled napkins and other excreta from the cubicle to avoid spread of infection, and a strict handwashing routine by all members of the ward team is essential. If the child is undergoing various tests then a short explanation should be given to explain the reason for not being allowed food or fluids and the child's co-operation in this can be obtained. If the test does not require the giving of a general anaesthetic then a nurse from the ward should accompany and stay with the child whilst the test is carried out, and taking a favourite doll or toy will also make the situation less frightening. If a child normally attends school or a play group then this should be continued in hospital so that the minimum disruption to daily living is experienced. When the child is ready for discharge the parents should be warned that he may take a little time to settle in at home and temper tantrums are not uncommon. There may also be some temporary regression in toilet training.

The premature baby

Congenital anomalies of the gastrointestinal tract may require urgent life-saving surgery to be carried out, and many babies admitted to a paediatric ward for this purpose are born prematurely. The nurse must appreciate that because of his prematurity this baby may not be able to control his temperature satisfactorily, and may suffer from respiratory difficulties as well. The premature baby is best nursed in an incubator where the temperature can be thermo-statically controlled (incubator temperature 32°C) and oxygen run into the cot at about 2–4 l per minute (this should only be given if the baby cannot maintain a satisfactory colour without additional oxygen). The humidity in the incubator can also be controlled and this will assist the respirations. Generally the baby only wears a napkin and lies on a disposable sheet so that complete freedom of movement is available. Nursing the baby in an incubator also provides a degree of isolation, but the nurse should always wear a gown and mask when handling the baby, and a strict handwashing routine must be enforced. Toilet care should consist of twice daily washing of the face and hands, the remainder of the body (except the buttocks) may be cleaned with a little warm olive oil, a bacteriostatic agent such as Phisohex or left alone. The buttocks must be washed and dried carefully each time the napkin is changed. Observations of the baby's temperature, pulse and respiratory rates may be recorded four hourly together with the number and type of stools passed, also the urinary output. The baby may be weighed in the cot or removed onto nursery scales provided the room is warm. Feeding may need to be at one, two or three hourly intervals depending on the size and condition of the baby. If the room is warm and the baby fit enough he may be well wrapped up and taken out of the cot for feeding, otherwise he should be supported in an upright position and fed in the incubator. Some feeds may need to be given by tube in order not to tire the baby unduly. Careful and constant observation of the baby is necessary, and he can be easily observed through the incubator. When the baby is bigger (about 2100 g) and well enough he may be dressed and removed to a warm nursery to continue his care, and this is now the time when the mother should be encouraged to spend part of the day with him learning to look after him. It is important that the new baby is deprived of his mother's attention for the shortest time possible, and that she gains confidence in handling him prior to discharge from hospital.

CHAPTER 14

Investigations of the Gastrointestinal Tract

In this chapter the preparation and after care of the patient will be considered in relation to certain investigations which may be carried out on the gastrointestinal tract. The reason for the various tests and the interpretation of the results obtained has already been described in the appropriate chapter.

The nurse must ensure that for all investigations the patient receives the appropriate preparation and arrives in the department in time and that the case notes and previous X-rays are available. The patient must be warmly dressed, have been able to pass urine before leaving the ward, and if expected to be away some little time has taken a book or morning paper with him. Where the investigation involves an X-ray the patient should wear a clean loose fitting gown closed by tapes and not metal fasteners. If the patient is away from the ward during a meal time the nurse must see that a suitable meal is given when the patient returns after completion of the test provided no anaesthetic has been given.

Sialography

A cannula is introduced into the openings of the parotid and submandibular ducts, iodized oil viscous injection (Lipiodol) is introduced into the ducts and an X-ray taken (sialogram). As this is an iodine preparation a test for iodine tolerance should be carried out prior to the investigation. No other specific treatment is required.

Augmented histamine test

The patient should fast for twelve hours. A Ryle's tube is passed and the gastric contents are aspirated. Aspiration continues for the next hour, either by continuous suction, or intermittent suction using a syringe. Thirty minutes after commencing this collection of gastric secretion mepyramine maleate (Anthisan) 50 mg is given by intramuscular injection. Thirty minutes later a subcutaneous injection of histamine acid phosphate 0·04 mg per kilo body weight is given and further collection of gastric juice continued as before for the next hour. The tube is then removed. The total volume of juice is measured and the total acid content of the secretion is estimated.

Pentagastrin test

The patient fasts for twelve hours. A Ryle's tube is passed into the stomach and the contents aspirated. Pentagastrin 6·0 g per kilo body weight is given as a subcutaneous injection which produces maximal stimulation after ten minutes. Aspiration of gastric contents continues at fifteen minute intervals for one hour after the injection. Side effects are minor and few. As an alternative the Pentagastrin (same dose) may be given in a slow intravenous infusion over a period of one hour.

Diagnex test

During the forty-eight hours prior to the investigation no medications should be given and this particularly includes iron preparations. The patient should fast for twelve hours. Betazole hydrochloride (Histalog) 50 mg or caffeine benzoate 500 mg is given orally. One hour later granules of Azure A (a dye) are given by mouth. Two hours later the urine is collected. If acid is being secreted in the stomach the urine should turn blue. Patients experience very few side effects.

Oesophagoscopy and gastroscopy

The patient should fast for twelve hours. An injection of atropine sulphate 0·5 mg is given forty-five minutes before the investigation, followed twenty minutes beforehand by a benzocaine compound lozenge 100 mg to suck. Some doctors prefer the patient to have an amethocaine gargle 1% shortly before the procedure is carried out. Diazepam (Valium) 5–10 mg may be given by slow intravenous injection immediately prior to passing the oesophagoscope to make the patient sleepy and the speech slurred. After the investigation has been completed no food or fluid should be given for at least three hours until the swallowing reflex has returned. If the patient experiences a sore throat then aspirin soluble tablets 1–3 (Disprin) may be given once feeding has recommenced.

Oesophagoscopy and gastroscopy in infants *see* Chapter 13.

Jejunal biopsy *see* Chapter 8 & Fig. 51.

Jejunal biopsy in infants *see* Chapter 13.

Colonoscopy

A flexible fibre-optic colonoscope is used for this investigation, and if only the sigmoid colon is to be examined then the patient may attend as an out-patient, but if a full colonoscopy to the caecum is required then the patient should be admitted for suitable preparation. For investigation of the sigmoid colon one enema is sufficient usually Veripaque 1 g in 500 ml and this is given one hour before the procedure. If a full colonoscopy is intended then the patient should have a low residue diet for two days and then a liquid diet immediately preceding the investigation. Castor oil 30 ml is given the afternoon before and a Veripaque enema 3 g in 1500 ml one hour before the procedure. This preparation ensures that the bowel is completely clean in 95% of patients. Diazepam (Valium) is given intravenously at the commencement of the procedure, and if it is expected to take a considerable while then a similar dose is given intramuscularly. A small dose of pethidine hydrochloride may be given intramuscularly. During the procedure the patient may be a little drowsy but able to cooperate and turn into a different position when required. The patient is allowed to rest for three or four hours after completion of the investigation and may be allowed home provided the journey is easy and he is escorted. Some patients complain of abdominal distension later, but the flatus is usually expelled quite quickly. Perforation of the gut is a possible, though fortunately rare complication.

Sigmoidoscopy

Preparation of the patient varies considerably from one surgeon to another, some requiring the patient to have an enema or washout the day before the examination, others prescribe bisacodyl (Dulcolax) suppositories to be given the day before, and some surgeons prefer no special preparation to be made. The investigation is carried out without the administration of an anaesthetic. A biopsy is often taken through the sigmoidoscope.

Sigmoidoscopy in infants *see* Chapter 13.

Investigations using barium

Barium swallow
The patient should not be given a meal immediately prior to the investigation. No other preparation is required except to warn the patient that the procedure is carried out in the dark.

Barium meal and follow through
The patient should not eat fruit or vegetables on the day prior to the investigation and all medicines are omitted for twenty-four hours.

An aperient such as Senokot 2 tablets is given twenty-four hours before the investigation, and should be repeated when all the X-rays have been taken. Nothing is given by mouth for the preceding six hours.

Barium enema

The patient should take a low residue diet without fruit and vegetables for forty-eight hours before the investigation. An aperient such as Senokot 2 tablets is given thirty-six hours and an enema saponis two hours beforehand. Probanthine 30 mg orally may be given one hour prior to the investigation.

Faecal fat estimation

A patient receiving between 50 and 150 g of fat a day in the diet (normal hospital diet) will excrete on average 3 or 4 g of fat daily in the faeces. When an abnormality exists as in steatorrhoea, the amount excreted on this diet will be 6 g or more each day. Where a more precise estimation is required then the patient should be given a diet containing 70 g fat daily, and the stools collected over a period of three days. Carmine markers may be given by mouth to indicate the start of the faecal collection. All faeces passed must be saved, a specimen of stool is insufficient.

Faecal fat estimation in infants *see* Chapter 13.

Needle biopsy of the liver

The preparation and care of the patient has been described in detail in Chapter 5.

Cholecystogram

An iodine sensitivity test should be carried out. A straight abdominal X-ray should be taken twenty-four hours after the patient has been given an aperient. Low residue meals are given on the day prior to the investigation, the last meal being at 19.00 hours. The patient is weighed and the dose of iopanoic acid (Telepaque) calculated. The Telepaque tablets or granules are given with water at 21.00 hours. No further food or fluid except sips of water is given until all X-rays are complete. The first of a series of X-rays will be taken next day at 09.00 hours. Telepaque is an iodine compound which is absorbed by the gut conveyed to the liver and secreted in the bile. When it reaches the gall bladder it undergoes concentration and is stored and therefore shows the gall bladder outline on an X-ray film.

Cholangiogram

This is a way of outlining the gall bladder and bile ducts by means of their blood vessels by the intravenous administration of the dye. Iodipamide meglumine (Biligrafin) is injected slowly over a period of ten minutes before the commencement of taking X-rays. As with the cholecystogram a sensitivity test should be done first.

T-tube cholangiogram

This investigation involves injection of iopanoic acid (Telepaque) directly into the common bile duct through a T-tube. This is usually done within a few days of operation for removal of the gall bladder with exploration of the common bile duct. No special preparation is necessary.

Tests involving radioactive isotopes

Schilling test

This test detects the absorption of vitamin B_{12}. The patient is not given breakfast if the test is to be carried out in the morning. Cobalt-58 (^{58}Co) 0·5 μCi labelled vitamin B_{12} is given orally at 10.00 hours. A complete twenty-four hours urine collection is made starting immediately after the dose is given. Two hours later an intramuscular injection of cyanocobalamin 1000 microgrammes is given. Minimal precautions are required when collecting the urine; the patient should retain his own urinal or bedpan, and the nurse should wear disposable gloves when transferring the urine carefully through a funnel into a suitable size container. No other precautions are necessary with regard to patient handling.

Liver scanning

The patient is given potassium perchlorate 400 mg orally two hours before the test and then he is taken to the radioisotope department where the whole procedure is carried out. An intravenous injection of technetium-99m (Tc^{99m}) labelled antimony sulphide 2 mCi is given, and fifteen minutes later the scan is carried out. Subsequently the urine is radioactive for forty-eight hours and the standard precautions must be taken if it is to be handled—this involves the use of a separate bedpan or urinal, the wearing of gloves when carefully disposing of the contents into the toilet and care in removing the gloves followed by handwashing. If urine is spilt it must be regarded as a major spill and the isotope physicist contacted immediately. In the meantime the area should be cordoned off so that no other object or person becomes contaminated. Wherever possible it is preferable if the patient can use the toilet direct. The half-life of technetium is extremely short and therefore it is safe to dispose of it in the normal sewage system since its radioactivity is minimal within twenty-four hours or so.

Index

Main references are given in bold type, figure references in italic